Preface

A PRACTICAL GU
ACCREDITATION IN LABORATORY
MEDICINE

David Burnett OBE, PhD, FRCPath
Formerly Consultant Clinical Biochemist to the St Albans and Hemel
Hempstead NHS Trust, UK
Consultant in Quality and Accreditation Systems

Editors:
Karen H Poyser, MSc, PhD, DipRCPath
Principal Biochemist, Clinical Biochemistry Department, Bronglais
General Hospital, Aberystwyth

Roy A Sherwood, MSc, DPhil
Consultant Biochemist, Clinical Biochemistry Department, King's College
Hospital, London

ACB VENTURE PUBLICATIONS

with generous support from BioRad Laboratories Ltd

ACKNOWLEDGEMENTS

The Author thanks the following organisations and individuals for permission to reproduce or adapt material for certain figures in this publication. In the case of some International Standards, the limitations imposed on reproduction of more than a fixed percentage of the document makes it essential to obtain the complete standard for study. In the text attention is drawn to the value of a number of International Standards and the reader is recommended to buy the full text of certain Standards, these are indicated (Appendix 2 Further reading) by an asterisk.

Extracts from British and International Standards are reproduced with the permission of BSI under licence number 2002SK/0274. Such publications can be obtained from BSI Customer Services, 389 Chiswick High Road, London W4 4AL (Tel + 44 (0) 20 8996 9001).

Permission to quote from standards and other material from Advisory, Conciliation and Arbitration Service (UK), Audit Commission (UK), BMJ Publishing Group London and Ross Anderson, Churchill Livingstone Edinburgh, Clinical Pathology Accreditation (UK) Ltd, Kogan Paul London, Medical Devices Agency (Department of Health UK), National Pathology Accreditation Advisory Council (Australia), Organization for Economic Co-operation and Development (OECD), Office of the Official Publications of the European Communities, Royal College of Pathologists (UK). Excerpts from the Health and Safety Executive documents are Crown Copyright and are reproduced with the permission of the Controller of HMSO. Full acknowledgement is made where appropriate in the text.

Thank you to Mr M J Hallworth, Department of Pathology, Royal Shrewsbury Hospital, UK for material used in Figure 9.22, to Chesterfield and North Derbyshire Royal Hospital NHS Trust, (Figure 9.8), to Dr Paul Tearle, PHLS, UK (Figure 10.9), Dr Ken Scott, New Cross Hospital, Wolverhampton (Figure 10.13) and to Mr G D Gogates (Figure 8.20).

Introduction and Contents

This book is intended to provide a practical guide to medical laboratories seeking external recognition for the quality of service they provide to their users. It uses two fictional devices to enable material of practical value to be presented to the reader. The first, an 'Ideal Standard' for medical laboratories is introduced in Chapter 3. Appendix 1 provides the structure of this standard and cross references to other important standards. It is recommended that the readers photocopy this appendix to use as a road map to the book. The second fictional device, is the Pathology Laboratory of St Elsewhere's Hospital Trust, which is introduced in Chapter 4 and from then on should become virtually a reality!

Chapter 1

Recognition of medical laboratories

INTRODUCTION

Medical laboratories seek recognition as being compliant with particular standards for a number of different reasons. In some countries it is mandatory and in others it may be voluntary. Even when it is voluntary, peer pressure or guidance on some aspect of healthcare from Government may indicate compliance with standards as being desirable. Reasons for seeking recognition range from a commercial imperative, such as it being a precondition for a contract, through to laboratory professionals wishing to practice in accordance with accepted norms.

There are a number of ways in which laboratories can seek recognition but the major choice is between accreditation and certification. This choice itself is confusing because, in common English usage, the two words have similar meanings. To *accredit* means 'to certify or guarantee someone or something as meeting required standards', and to *certify* means 'to endorse or guarantee that certain required standards have been met'.

However, within the International Organization for Standardization (ISO), the words have specific technical meanings. The definitions for this technical usage are given in Figure 1.1.

---

accreditation
procedure by which an authoritative body gives formal recognition that a body or person is competent to carry out specific tasks.

certification
procedure by which a third party gives written assurance that a product, process or service conforms to specific requirements.

ISO/IEC Guide 2 General terms and their definitions concerning standardization and related activity

---

Figure 1.1 ISO definitions of accreditation and certification

The distinction between the two activities will become clearer in Chapter 2 when the standards upon which accreditation or certification activities are based are discussed. Briefly, certification activity is based upon standards such as ISO 9001:2000 which delineate the 'requirements for quality management systems' and are applicable to any activity. Accreditation systems are based on standards that, in addition to 'requirements for quality systems', have so called 'technical requirements' that relate to achieving competence in all aspects of laboratory activity. However, standards for quality management systems, such as ISO 9001:2000 have a major impact upon the structure and content of standards used for laboratory accreditation. This chapter looks at what accreditation is, why it is needed and how it works.

WHAT IS ACCREDITATION?

DEFINITION AND CHARACTERISTICS
A useful definition of accreditation in relation to healthcare is given in Figure 1.2. The words in italics bring out the main characteristics of accreditation systems. In the early development of accreditation systems, professionals come together *voluntarily* to formulate a set of *standards* that are seen as representing current views on good practice. An important part of the activity is seen as educational, and facilities (medical laboratories) *voluntarily* agree to be assessed or measured against the standards. If a facility is seen to be in *substantial compliance* with the standards, then within the professional framework appropriate *recognition* is given.

Accreditation in healthcare....

'Professional and national *recognition* reserved for facilities that provide *quality* healthcare. This means that the particular healthcare facility has *voluntarily* sought to be *measured* against high professional *standards* and is in *substantial compliance* with them'

Anon

Figure 1.2 A definition of accreditation in healthcare

The initial impetus for establishing hospital or laboratory accreditation systems in a country commonly comes from healthcare professionals themselves, motivated at best by a concern for standards of patient care, or at least by enlightened self interest. During the initial development of accreditation systems, government agencies sometimes provide financial support or seek observer status. This stage is almost inevitably followed by some regulatory activity. Political expediency seems to determine the speed with which governments act, and is generally in response to some level of public concern or to a desire to regulate public expenditure on healthcare.

In countries where the conduct of laboratory medicine becomes increasingly subject to legislation, some of the voluntary and educational aspects of accreditation can too easily be displaced by an emphasis on inspection and compliance. However, governments will often recognise the work of originating organizations, such as the College of American Pathologists (CAP), as accrediting bodies, thus preserving the valuable contribution that such agencies make to quality improvement within a statutory context.

SCOPE OF ACCREDITATION
In healthcare organizations accreditation can recognise a number of different activities (Figure 1.3).

Accreditation can recognise.....

- the competence of a person to carry out specified tasks

- a healthcare facility, or post in that facility, as suitable for training

- a healthcare facility as having reached the standard required to perform a prescribed function

---

Figure 1.3 Scope of accreditation

In many countries there are well established mechanisms for recognising training posts in medical laboratories and a burgeoning interest in monitoring the ongoing competence of individuals to perform in their chosen profession. In the past, training and competence of professionals has always had a part in establishing that a particular laboratory has reached a requisite standard for its prescribed function. Current concerns in many parts of the world about the quality of laboratory services will increase the focus on all these aspects of accreditation.

WHY IS ACCREDITATION NEEDED?

For a laboratory to seek accreditation is to acknowledge that being in compliance with recognised standards is important (Figure 1.4). The fundamental reasons for a laboratory being accredited are the same whether it is in the private or public sector or whether accreditation is mandatory or voluntary. If the laboratory is in the private sector, the commercial imperative is to be recognised as operating in compliance with high standards. Similarly, those laboratories in the public sector acting as referral laboratories (external laboratories to which a sample is submitted for a supplementary or confirmatory examination procedure and report) benefit from a similar confirmation.

Accreditation is important because it....

- recognises competence

- facilitates exchange of services

- provides a valuable management tool

- ensures that the needs and requirements of all users (clinicians and patients) are met

Figure 1.4 Importance of accreditation

For laboratory professionals who seek to work in a professional manner, it is essential to have this competence recognised in the accreditation process (Figure 1.5). The emerging generation of standards, with their emphasis on quality management and continual improvement, provides the opportunity for creative and innovative ways of working. They demand a constant review of where you are and where you want to be, and assist in ensuring that the needs and requirements of users are met.

'It is in the interests of patients, of society, and of governments that clinical laboratories operate at high standards of professional and technical competence...
It is in the interests of competent laboratories that their competence is verified through a process of inspection, comparison against appropriate standards, as a confirmation of their good standing... Adherence to high standards, such as those related to timeliness of test results, laboratory accuracy and precision, clinical relevance of the tests performed, qualifications and training of personnel and prevention of errors, is an ethical responsibility of all clinical laboratory staff'

extracts from Principles of Clinical Laboratory Accreditation
A policy statement by IFCC and WASP (1999)

Figure 1.5 Principles of laboratory accreditation

HOW DOES ACCREDITATION WORK ?

ELEMENTS OF AN ACCREDITATION SYSTEM
In my book, 'Understanding Accreditation in Laboratory Medicine', an accreditation system was described as having three elements, the accreditation authority or body, the inspectors or assessors, and the standards. In countries where accredi-

tation is mandatory, accreditation bodies have their constituency (the laboratories to be accredited) defined in legislation; in these countries there is no choice for laboratories but to be part of an accreditation system. In countries where accreditation is voluntary, laboratories have a choice as to whether to participate or not, and in a sense, can be described as being the fourth element of an accreditation system. Even when participation is compulsory it is important that accreditation bodies maintain a dialogue with the laboratories. The four elements are defined in Figure 1.6.

The **ACCREDITATION BODY** which oversees the assessments and grants accreditation (and may also set the standards)

The **STANDARDS** with which a laboratory has to comply in order to gain accreditation

The **ASSESSORS or inspectors** who seek to establish compliance with the standards by conducting the assessment

The **USER LABORATORY** which is required to, or voluntarily seeks to, comply with the standards by being assessed

---

Figure 1.6 Elements of an accreditation system

Some accreditation bodies set standards and others use standards set by national or international standards organizations. Their main task is to oversee assessments of laboratories against the standards and to grant or refuse accreditation on the basis of compliance or noncompliance. There are international standards and guides that set requirements for accreditation bodies themselves, and for the assessments they oversee. The standards used in accreditation systems will be discussed in the next chapter.

DIFFERENT MODELS
The way in which accreditation has evolved in different countries determines the way in which accreditation systems and the bodies that run them have developed. Accreditation bodies are of two distinct types, those formed by professional organizations (which can operate at provincial, national or, occasionally, at an international level), and those recognised by national government to have responsibility for accreditation (National Accreditation bodies). Examples of the former are Clinical Pathology Accreditation (UK) Ltd (CPA) in the United Kingdom, and Coordinatie Commissie voor Kwaliteitsbewaking in Laboratatoria in de gezondheidszorg (CCKLTest) in The Netherlands. In the UK the corresponding National

Accreditation body is the United Kingdom Accreditation Service (UKAS), and in The Netherlands, Raad voor Accreditatie (RvA). In both countries accreditation is voluntary.

In The Netherlands, CCKLTest works closely with RvA for inspector training whilst still retaining operational independence. Medical laboratories that need to perform tests for international customers are accredited through RvA on a joint basis with CCKLTest. In the United Kingdom, CPA has signed a declaration of intent to co-operate with the UKAS but operates independently. It derives its authority from the shareholding membership of its management board, which includes observers from the UK Departments of Health, and from its wide acceptance by laboratories in the National Health Service (NHS) and the private sector.

In the USA, accreditation is mandatory and the standards to be met are enshrined in the Clinical Laboratory Improvement Amendments of 1988 (CLIA'88) Act. Inspection can be carried out by the Centers for Medicare and Medicaid Services (formerly the Healthcare Financing Administration), or by organizations recognised under the act as 'deemed authorities' such as the College of American Pathologists and the Joint Commission on Accreditation of Healthcare Organizations. These deemed authorities set their own standards, which can include requirements over and above those required by CLIA'88.

In Sweden and South Africa, the medical laboratory professionals have developed close working relationships with their respective National Accreditation bodies, SWEDAC and SANAS, and their inspectors undertake assessments together with appropriately qualified laboratory professionals.

INTERNATIONAL AND REGIONAL GROUPINGS
At international level, the International Laboratory Accreditation Co-operation (ILAC) is the principal forum for the development of laboratory accreditation practices and procedures. It facilitates a uniform approach to determining laboratory competence through accreditation and sees this as leading to mutual recognition agreements between countries that enhance and facilitate the international acceptance of test data and eliminate technical barriers to trade. It also provides assistance to countries that are in the process of establishing their own accreditation systems. In conjunction with ILAC, specific regions have established their own co-operations. For example, in the Asia-Pacific region, the Asia-Pacific Laboratory Accreditation Co-operation (APLAC), in the Americas, the InterAmerican Accreditation Co-operation (IAAC) and in Europe, the European Co-operation for Accreditation (EA). EA is mandated by the European Community to look after matters affecting accreditation in the Community.

Chapter 2

The changing world of standards

INTRODUCTION

In the first chapter the nature of accreditation was explained, in particular that accreditation systems are based on standards that have requirements for both quality management and technical competence. In this chapter the nature of standards and their development is examined and standards of value in the medical laboratory are introduced.

STANDARDS, GUIDELINES, PRINCIPLES OR CRITERIA

WHAT IS A STANDARD?

The use of the word 'standard' requires some explanation. In science and technology it is described as having two different meanings, the first as a 'normative document' and the second as a 'measurement standard'. Its use to mean a measurement standard is used in the context of laboratory examinations or analysis. Normative in the context of the term normative document means 'implying, creating or prescribing a norm or standard'. A definition of a standard as a normative document is given in Figure 2.1. These normative documents contain a number of titled clauses which are the requirements of the standard.

---

standard
document, established by consensus and approved by a recognized body, that provides, for common and repeated use, rules, guidelines or characteristics for activities or their results, aimed at the achievement of the optimum degree of order in a given context

ISO/IEC Guide 2 General terms and their definition concerning standardization and related activities

---

Figure 2.1 A definition of a standard as a normative document

Examples of such normative documents are the International Standards published by the International Organization for Standardization*, ISO 17025:1999 'General requirements for the competence of testing and calibration laboratories' and ISO 9001:2000 'Quality management systems – Requirements'.

When the term 'international standard' is used in lower case it signifies a document adopted by an international standards organization, but not ISO. Where it is in upper and lower case, i.e.'International Standard', it is an international standard created by ISO or the International Electrotechnical Commission (IEC).

Apart from this technical use of the word standard as a normative document it is also used in other accreditation systems to mean 'an accepted or approved example of something against which others are judged'. In such systems, the laboratory is assessed against 'a standard document' that contains a number of standards that are equivalent to the clauses in a normative document. Other accreditation systems use documents which describe guidelines, principles or criteria as the basis for assessment. In common English usage all these words are defined by reference to the word 'standard'.

WHY DO WE NEED STANDARDS?
The effectiveness of any accreditation system is crucially dependent on the standards adopted and on the objectivity of assessment of compliance. The requirement for standards arises from the description of accreditation as recognition 'for facilities that provide quality healthcare' (Figure 1.2) and from the importance of accreditation to a medical laboratory (Figure 1.4). Standards are required which reflect a quest for quality and promote harmonization of practice from laboratory to laboratory and from country to country. For a person with diabetes, who moves from place to place, and perhaps from country to country, the quality of the measurement of HbA1c will have long term implications for their healthcare outcome.

QUALITY
Before trying to assess quality or measure compliance with standards which purport to represent quality, it is important to attempt a definition of quality. Within ISO and elsewhere there have been many attempts to define quality and the latest of a long line of ISO definitions is given in Figure 2.2.

---

* ISO is a term derived from the Greek isosos meaning 'equal' and is the root of the prefix used in many terms such as 'isometric' (of equal measure or dimensions). From 'equal' to 'standard' the line of thinking led to ISO being used as the name of the organization to avoid the plethora of acronymns which would have resulted from translating the title of the organization into different languages.

---

quality
degree to which a set of inherent characteristics fulfils requirements

ISO 9000:2000 Quality management systems – Fundamentals and vocabulary

---

Figure 2.2 ISO definition of quality

This sort of definition is almost impenetrable to those not familiar with the world of standards, but relating it to a clinical situation can help to bring it to life. For example, a patient in a hypoglycaemic coma has a 'requirement' for a blood glucose measurement and the 'inherent characteristics' of that measurement are that it be done on the correct specimen in an accurate and timely manner and be properly interpreted in order to provide a quality result or service.

HARMONIZATION AND SUBSIDIARITY

In order to have harmonization of practice in any field of endeavour it is necessary to create a standard against which practice can be measured. ISO, in its mission statement, defines its task as 'promoting the development of standardization and related activities in the world with a view to facilitating the international exchange of goods and services and to develop co-operation in the fields of intellectual, scientific, technological and economic activity'. Harmonization of practice requires mechanisms with which to introduce, apply and monitor standards. This is the role of accreditation bodies, which were described in the previous chapter.

Although harmonization of practice in medical laboratories is important there is more than one way to achieve this goal. In the European Community, the principle of subsidiarity requires the Community to act; 'only if and so far as the objectives of the proposed action cannot be sufficiently achieved by Member States, and can therefore, by reason of the scale or the effects of the proposed action, be better achieved by the Community'. Subsidiarity in its original philosophical meaning* of being 'concerned with fostering social responsibility' can be translated as saying that architects of standards and of accreditation schemes must be wary of aggregating to themselves rights which may not be acceptable to the 'fourth element of accreditation', the laboratories to be accredited.

---

* The principle of subsidiarity in its original philosophical meaning was expressed by Pope Pius XI in his Encyclical letter in 1931; 'It is an injustice, a grave evil and disturbance of right order for a larger and higher association to arrogate to itself functions which can be performed efficiently by smaller and lower sections'.

Different situations require different solutions. In countries with limited resources or where accreditation is voluntary, benefit can be gained from development of standards or guidelines for national use and this principle of subsidiarity can then be seen as promoting the long term aim of harmonization.

HOW ARE STANDARDS DEVELOPED?

PROCESS

The way in which standards (normative documents) are developed has much in common irrespective of the organization involved. The ISO develops its standards according to the principles shown in Figure 2.3.

CONSENSUS
the views of all interests are taken into account: manufacturers, vendors and users consumer groups, testing laboratories

INDUSTRY-WIDE
global solutions to satisfy industries and customers worldwide

VOLUNTARY
international standardization is market-driven and therefore based on voluntary involvement of all interests in the market place

International Organization for Standardization (ISO)

Figure 2.3 Principles for development of ISO standards

There are three main phases in the development of an ISO standard. When a need for an International Standard is expressed by a particular sector, such as the medical laboratory community, it is normally communicated via a National Standards body, such as the British Standards Institution in the United Kingdom, to ISO as a whole. Once the need has been agreed the first phase involves the definition of the scope of the standard and the work is carried out in a working group comprising technical experts from interested countries.

Once agreement is reached on the scope of the standard, the second phase, the consensus building begins. During this phase the detailed specifications within the standard are negotiated. The final phase comprises the formal approval of the resulting draft International Standard following which the agreed text is published.

STRUCTURE AND DRAFTING

The detailed rules for the structure and drafting of an International Standard are given in ISO/IEC Directives, Part 2. It has normative and informative elements. The normative elements describe the scope of the standard and set out its provisions. These provisions can be expressed as requirements, recommendations or statements (Figure 2.4).

---

requirement
expression in the content of a document conveying criteria to be fulfilled if compliance with the document is to be claimed and from which no deviation is permitted

recommendation
expression in the content of a document conveying that among several possibilities one is recommended as particularly suitable, without mentioning or excluding others, or that a certain course of action is preferred but not necessarily required, or that (in the negative form) a certain possibility or course of action is deprecated but not prohibited

statement
expression in the content of a document conveying information

based on ISO/IEC Directives, Part 2, 2001

Figure 2.4 ISO definitions for provisions

Requirements are expressed using the verbal form 'shall' and recommendations using 'should'. Statements indicating a course of action permissible within the document use the verbal form 'may' and statements of possibility and capability use 'can'.

Informative elements can be preliminary or supplementary. Preliminary elements are those that identify the document, introduce its content and explain its background, its development and its relationship with other documents. Supplementary elements provide additional information intended to assist with the understanding or use of the document.

Figure 2.5 indicates these different elements with reference to the International Standard, ISO 17025:1999 'General requirements for the competence of testing and calibration laboratories'.

Title page **(Title)**	Informative **(Normative)**
Contents	Informative
Foreword	Informative
Introduction	Informative
Title	**Normative**
1 Scope	**Normative**
2 Normative references	**Normative**
3 Terms and definitions	**Normative**
4 Management requirements	**Normative**
5 Technical requirements	**Normative**
Annex A Nominal cross reference to ISO 9001:1994 and ISO 9002:1994	Informative
Annex B Guidelines for establishing applications for specific fields	Informative
Bibliography	Informative

Figure 2.5 The normative and informative elements of ISO 17025:1999

Within a standard document there are rules concerning the hierachy of clauses, sub-clauses, paragraphs and lists. Clauses create the basic sub-division and are continuously numbered with Arabic numerals beginning with 1 for the 'Scope' clause through to, but not including, any annexes (see Figure 2.5). Each clause has a title.

Sub-clauses can be primary, e.g. 4.1, secondary, e.g. 4.1.1 and, if necessary, through to the fifth level (e.g. 4.1.1.1.1.1). Primary sub-clauses should preferably be given a title and secondary sub-clauses may be treated in the same way. A paragraph is an unnumbered sub-division of a clause or sub-clause. Lists may be used within a clause or sub-clause and introduced by a sentence, e.g. 'The procedure(s) adopted shall ensure that'; and completed by items of the list preceded by a dash, bullet, or for ease of identification, by a lower case letter e.g. a). These rules are illustrated in Figure 2.6 with material from ISO 15189:2002.

4 Management requirements   **Main clause**

4.1 Organization and management   **Primary sub-clause**

4.1.1   The laboratory or the organization of which it is   **Secondary sub-clauses**
        a part shall be legally identifiable

4.1.2   Medical laboratory...........

4.1.5   The laboratory management shall have
        responsibility for the design, implementation and
        maintenance of the quality management system.
        This shall include:

        a) management support of all laboratory personnel by   **List**
           providing them with the appropriate authority and
           resources to carry out their duties;
        b) have arrangements to ensure that its management
           and personnel are free from undue internal...;
        c) policies and procedures to ensure the protection of
           confidential information....

        based on ISO 15189:2002 Medical laboratories – Particular requirements for quality and competence

Figure 2.6 ISO clauses, sub-clauses, paragraphs and lists

CONTENT

The different elements of an International Standard were shown in Figure 2.5. A careful study of the preliminary informative elements is important, in particular the foreword and introduction, as this is where valuable information such as its intended use, can be found. Nothing presented in the foreword or introduction must be regarded as a requirement of the standard. The title of an International Standard is important and needs to convey as clearly as possible the nature of the standard. It is well illustrated by the change in title of ISO 15189 during its development from, 'Quality management in the medical laboratory' to 'Medical laboratories – Particular requirements for quality and competence'.

The first numbered normative element is the **scope**. This is intended to define, without ambiguity, the subject of the document and the aspects of the topic covered. The scope indicates the applicability of the document. As we shall see when introducing standards of value to medical laboratories the scope can be brief or extensive. The second normative element is **normative references**. This is an optional element, but when it is present the references are almost invariably to other ISO standards. If a standard is referenced in this section, the implication is that it is indispensable to the application of the document, to the extent that compliance with the document signifies compliance with the content of the standard cited.

The third element **terms and definitions** is also optional but, if used, provides the technical sense in which particular terms are used in the document. It can include a term and definition or refer to other ISO Standards which define terms. It is prefaced by the phrase 'For the purposes of this document, the terms given in (reference to Standard).... and the following apply'. Key sources of terms and definitions relevant to this book are found in the references shown in Figure 2.7.

ISO 9000:2000	Quality management systems – Fundamentals and vocabulary
ISO/IEC Guide 2	General terms and their definitions concerning standardization and related activities
VIM	International vocabulary of basic and general terms in metrology, issued by BIPM, IEC, IFCC, ISO, IUPAC, IUPAP and OIML
ISO 14050:1998	Environmental management – Vocabulary

Figure 2.7 Sources of terms and definitions

The elements which follow the terms and definitions, are the main clauses that contain the **provisions** of the standard. As shown in Figure 2.4 these can be in the form of requirements, recommendations or statements. Finally there follows optional informative, or occasionally, normative elements in Annexes and a Bibliography.

STANDARDS FOR MEDICAL LABORATORIES

Standards of value to medical laboratories concern both quality and competence. The concept of quality in relation to the need for standards has been briefly mentioned earlier in this chapter. In Chapter 3 this emphasis on quality and competence is examined in relation to the role and function of medical laboratories.

Until the recent publication of the document, ISO/IEC 15189:2002 'Medical laboratories – Particular requirements for quality and competence' there were no sector specific ISO standards for quality management and technical competence in medical laboratories. There are two distinct lines of International Standard development applicable to the medical laboratory.

The first line focuses on the 'requirements for quality management systems' applicable to any organization, represented by ISO 9001:2000 and a second line, with its origin in assessing the technical competence of laboratories, is represented by ISO 17025:1999, a generic standard used in the accreditation of any type of testing or calibration laboratory and the sector specific standard ISO 15189:2002 for medical laboratories. These main reference sources are shown in Figure 2.8 together with their application and abbreviations used in this book.

Title of the standard	Application	Abbreviation used in text
ISO 9001:2000 Quality management systems – Requirements	For quality system management	ISO 9001:2000
ISO/IEC 17025:1999 General requirements for the competence of testing and calibration laboratories	For quality and competence of testing and calibration laboratories	ISO 17025:1999
ISO/IEC 15189:2002 Medical laboratories – Particular requirements for quality and competence	For quality and competence of medical laboratories	ISO 15189:2002

Figure 2.8   Standards used as main reference sources

It is important to commit to memory the abbreviations (and corresponding application information) shown in Figure 2.8 as they will be used throughout the book.

ISO 9001:2000 QUALITY MANAGEMENT SYSTEMS – REQUIREMENTS
This standard is one of a family of related quality management system standards shown in Figure 2.9, all of which will have an increasingly important role in defining quality management and continual improvement in the medical laboratory.

The standard specifies requirements for an organization, such as a medical laboratory, wishing to establish an effective quality management system that embraces the concept of continual improvement and to demonstrate its ability to consistently provide a product that meets the users needs. In the case of a medical laboratory this product, better thought of as a service, is represented by consultative, examination and interpretative activity that results in the issuing of a report. Different aspects of the **scope** of the standard are discussed in detail in Chapter 3.

Title of the standard	Abbreviation used in text
ISO 9000:2000 Quality management systems – Fundamentals and vocabulary	ISO 9000:2000
ISO 9001:2000 Quality management systems – Requirements	**ISO 9001:2000**
ISO 9004:2000 Quality management systems – Guidelines for performance improvement	ISO 9004:2000

Figure 2.9 The ISO quality management systems family of standards

It is important to note that ISO 9001:2000 does not provide specifications for the report (product or service) itself, nor the requirements for assessing the (technical) competence of the laboratory to undertake the pre-examination, examination and post-examination processes necessary to produce the report. The titles of the main clauses and primary sub-clauses that encompass the provisions of the standard are shown in Figure 2.10.

ISO 17025:1999 GENERAL REQUIREMENTS FOR THE COMPETENCE OF TESTING AND CALIBRATION LABORATORIES
The introduction to this International Standard contains two statements of importance to those laboratories making the choice between pursuing certification and/or accreditation. It states that testing and calibration laboratories that comply with ISO 17025:1999 will also operate in accordance with ISO 9001:2000, but goes on to remind the reader that certification against ISO 9001:2000 does not demonstrate the competence of the laboratory to produce technically valid data and results. The scope of this International Standard includes a number of key issues that are summarised in Figure 2.11.

4 Quality management system
4.1 General requirements
4.2 Documentation requirements

5 Management responsibility
5.1 Management commitment
5.2 Customer focus
5.3 Quality policy
5.4 Planning
5.5 Management review

6 Resource management
6.1 Provision of resources
6.2 Human resources
6.3 Infrastructure
6.4 Work environment

7 Product realization
7.1 Planning of product realization
7.2 Customer-related processes
7.3 Design and development
7.4 Purchasing
7.5 Production and service provision
7.6 Control of monitoring and measuring devices

8 Measurement, analysis and improvement
8.1 General
8.2 Monitoring and measurement
8.3 Control of nonconforming product
8.4 Analysis of data
8.5 Improvement

Figure 2.10 The requirements of ISO 9001:2000

The scope of ISO 17025:1999...

• specifies the general requirements for the competence to carry out tests and/or calibrations, including sampling. It covers standard, non-standard and laboratory-developed methods

• is applicable to all testing/calibration laboratories regardless of the number of personnel or extent of the scope of its activities

• is for use by laboratories developing their quality, administrative and technical systems that govern their operations

• is for use by laboratory clients, regulatory authorities and accreditation bodies who wish to confirm or recognise the competence of laboratories

• does not cover compliance with regulatory and safety requirements for the operation of laboratories

Figure 2.11 The scope of ISO 17025:1999

The titles of the main clauses and primary sub-clauses of ISO 17025:1999 are given in Figure 2.12 together with those of the sector specific standard for medical laboratories, ISO 15189:2002 for comparison.

ISO 17025:1999	ISO 15189:2002
4 Management requirements	**4 Management requirements**
4.1 Organization	4.1 Organization and management
4.2 Quality system	4.2 Quality management system
4.3 Document control	4.3 Document control
4.4 Review of requests, tenders and contracts	4.4 Review of contracts
4.5 Sub-contracting of tests and calibrations	4.5 Examination by referral laboratories
4.6 Purchasing supplies and services	4.6 External supplies and services
4.7 Service to the client	4.7 Advisory services
4.8 Complaints	4.8 Resolution of complaints
4.9 Control of nonconforming testing and/or calibration work	4.9 Identification and control of nonconformities
4.10 Corrective action	4.10 Corrective action
4.11 Preventative action	4.11 Preventative action
	4.12 Continual improvement
4.12 Control of records	4.13 Quality and technical records
4.13 Internal audits	4.14 Internal audits
4.14 Management review	4.15 Management review
5 Technical requirements	**5 Resources and technical requirements**
5.1 General	
5.2 Personnel	5.1 Personnel
5.3 Accommodation and environmental conditions	5.2 Accommodation and environmental conditions
5.4 Test and method validation	5.5 Examination procedures
5.5 Equipment	5.3 Laboratory equipment
5.6 Measurement traceability	
5.7 Sampling	5.4 Pre-examination procedures
5.8 Handling of test and calibration items	
5.9 Assuring the quality of test and calibration results	5.6 Assuring the quality of examination procedures
5.10 Reporting results	5.7 Post-examination procedures <u>and</u>
	5.8 Reporting results

Figure 2.12 The provisions of ISO 17025:1999 and ISO 15189:2002

ISO 15189:2002 MEDICAL LABORATORIES – PARTICULAR REQUIREMENTS FOR QUALITY AND COMPETENCE

The **scope** clause of this International Standard is very brief, but by bringing together aspects of the foreword and introduction it is possible to develop this into a proposal for an extended statement of scope as shown in Figure 2.13.

An extended scope for ISO 15189:1999...

- specifies particular requirements for the quality and competence of medical laboratories

- covers all examinations and provides guidance for laboratory procedures to ensure quality in medical laboratory examinations

- is applicable to all currently recognized disciplines of medical laboratory services

- is for use by medical laboratories developing the quality, administrative and technical systems that govern their operation

- is based upon the normative documents ISO 17025:1999 and ISO 9001:2000 and these documents, plus the corresponding tables in Appendix A, are an integral part of this International Standard

- is for use by bodies who wish to confirm or recognise the competence of medical laboratories

---

Figure 2.13 A proposed extended scope for ISO 15189:2002

OTHER REFERENCE SOURCES

The main references described above contain general requirements for quality and competence. Although ISO 15189:2002 is entitled 'Medical laboratories – Particular requirements for quality and competence', the word particular is used relative to medical laboratories. The standard is still general/generic in the sense that it is applicable to all currently recognised disciplines in pathology.

In addition to these standards there are many other sources of standards and guidelines of value in medical laboratories. These can be usefully divided into materials which are a) national standards or guidelines, e.g. CPA(UK)Ltd Standards for the Medical Laboratory (2001), b) discipline-specific, e.g. Standards for Histocompat-ability Testing, European Federation for Immunogenetics (1999) or c) topic-specific, e.g. Retention of laboratory records and diagnostic material, National Pathology Accreditation Advisory Council, (2001). These will be included together with useful websites in Appendix 2 Further reading.

It is also important to remember that, even in countries where there is no legislation governing accreditation, often a standard, or explanatory information associated with the standard, points to a requirement to comply with national, regional and international regulations and legislation.

Chapter 3

Quality management for the medical laboratory

INTRODUCTION

The first two chapters discussed the nature of accreditation and the standards which underpin accreditation systems. Accreditation is not about getting a 'designer' label for the laboratory, it is about putting standards into practice and using them to manage quality and continual improvement in medical laboratories.

In Chapter 2, two distinct lines of International Standard development applicable to the medical laboratory were identified. The first focused on the 'requirements for quality management systems' applicable to any organization or activity, represented by the ISO family of standards. The second line, with its origin in assessing the technical competence of laboratories, is represented by ISO 17025:1999, a generic standard used in the accreditation of any type of testing laboratory and the sector specific standard, ISO 15189:2002 'Medical Laboratories – Particular requirements for quality and technical competence'. The use of the term 'technical competence' in the title is best read as 'competence' as the scope is much broader than use of the word 'technical' would imply in the context of a medical laboratory.

The latter standards contain requirements for (quality) management, but their presentation in a separate section from the technical (competence) requirements does not enable the user to see easily how the two can be integrated. This chapter will create a framework within which these two sets of requirements can be integrated. As this framework is developed the structure of a new standard for use in the accreditation of medical laboratories will emerge and be presented in language which will hopefully be acceptable to the medical laboratory community, whilst preserving the principles of International Standard development. In this book it will be called the 'Ideal Standard'.

QUALITY AND COMPETENCE

In Chapter 2 quality was defined as the 'degree to which a set of inherent characteristics fulfils requirements' and an attempt was made to translate this into terms familiar to medical laboratory professionals. Another approach to quality in medical laboratories is to examine whether the laboratory is 'fit for its purpose'. An immediate consequence of this approach is the need to define the purpose of a medical laboratory service. This is perhaps an appropriate subject for a complete book, but a useful working definition was published by the Department of Health (UK) in 1970 (Figure 3.1).

'To provide a consultant advisory service supported by adequate scientific diagnostic facilities in the laboratory, at the bedside, in the outpatient department and in the home, covering all aspects of laboratory investigation including the interpretation of results and advice on further appropriate investigation'

Department of Health, United Kingdom HM(70)60 August 1970

Figure 3.1 The purpose of a medical laboratory service

In order to achieve this purpose a laboratory needs to manage quality in all aspects of its organization and to ensure the competence of the organization and of the individuals who work within it.

Although the word competence appears in the title of both the laboratory standards, ISO 17025:1999 and ISO 15189:2002 (Figure 2.8), it is not formally defined in either document. In the context of these standards it refers to the ability of a laboratory (organization) to perform specified tasks. The ISO definition of 'competence' is a 'demonstrated ability to apply knowledge and skills'. This implies that, in addition to an organization or person having the ability to apply knowledge and skills to a particular task, there must be some objective test to substantiate this ability. For example, in order to become an auditor, ISO/DIS 19011:2002 'Guidelines on the quality and/or environmental management systems', states that 'a person should have appropriate personal attributes and demonstrate an ability to apply appropriate knowledge and skills' (see Chapter 11). Education, training and experience being the means by which these can be acquired.

It follows that for a laboratory (an organization) to be seen as competent, it will need attributes relevant to its task (see Chapter 4), knowledgeable and skillful personnel (see Chapter 6), appropriate premises, equipment etc. (see Chapters 7 and 8) and be able to demonstrate effective examination processes (see Chapters 9 and 10).

PROCESS-BASED QUALITY MANAGEMENT

The starting point for developing a framework for process-based quality management of a medical laboratory and an 'Ideal Standard' lies in the introduction to ISO 9001:2000. It promotes the adoption of 'a process approach when developing, implementing and improving the effectiveness of a quality management system' in order 'to enhance customer satisfaction by meeting customer requirements'. Process is described as 'an activity using resources, managed in order to enable the transformation of inputs into outputs'. In the context of a medical laboratory, this may be 'consultation with users, receiving a request for an examination, carrying out the work and reporting the results, with interpretation where appropriate'.

Within any organization (e.g. a medical laboratory) there are numerous inter-related or interacting processes, and it is 'the identification and interactions of these processes and their management', that is referred to as a 'process approach'. It is the adoption of this approach that creates a process-based quality management system. Figure 3.2 below, adapted from ISO 9001:2000, represents a model of such a system. The numbers *4-8* in the figure correspond to the main clauses of ISO 9001:2000 (see Figure 2.10).

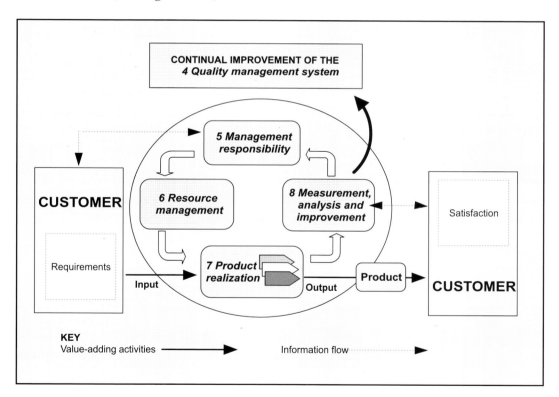

Figure 3.2 Model of a process-based quality management system (adapted from ISO 9001:2000)

In looking at this model it is helpful to translate some of the terms used into language more familiar to medical laboratory professionals. It can be viewed in two different ways. Firstly, the user (customer) has requirements that are formulated in consultation with laboratory management (5 Management responsibility) and the laboratory responds by carrying out pre-examination, examination and post-examination processes (7 Product realization) to produce a report (product) for the user. Depending on whether their requirements have been met or not, users may be defined as 'satisfied' or 'dissatisfied'. The second view, is that of a process model in which laboratory management (5 Management responsibility) creates a quality system (4 Quality management system) and uses resources, staff, equipment etc. (6 Resource management) to carry out pre-examination, examination and post-examination processes (7 Product realization) to fulfil the requirements of the user. The pre-examination, examination and post-examination processes are continually evaluated and improvements made as appropriate (8 Measurement, analysis and improvement). Evaluation and continual improvement activities would include for example, assessment of users needs and requirements, internal audit of the examination processes and review of participation in external quality assessment schemes.

PRINCIPLES OF QUALITY MANAGEMENT

The introduction of ISO 9000:2000 (Figure 2.9) puts forward the eight quality management principles identified as being of value to (laboratory) management in leading an organization towards improved performance. These principles are enumerated in Figure 3.3 and will be further discussed in this chapter and in later sections of the book.

• Customer focus	• System approach to management
• Leadership	• Continual improvement
• Involvement of people	• Factual decision making
• Process approach	• Mutually beneficial supplier

Figure 3.3 Principles of quality management

TOWARDS A PROCESS-BASED 'IDEAL STANDARD'

The purpose of creating an 'Ideal Standard' for this book is two-fold. Firstly to have a standard written in user friendly language and secondly, to provide a framework through which the standards can come off the paper and become part of the living reality of the laboratory services. All the sample documentation created throughout the book will follow the structure of the 'Ideal Standard'. The concept of an 'Ideal Standard' is not far from reality as a decision has already been made in principle within the appropriate ISO committees, to realign ISO 17025:1999 and ISO 15189:2002 with the structure of ISO 9001:2000.

In Figure 3.4 the correspondance between the main clauses of ISO 9001:2000 and the proposed 'Ideal Standard' is shown. Where the clause titles in ISO 9001:2000 are readily understood they are retained, but others are translated into more familiar terms. For example, the use of the terms 'measurement and analysis' in the title of the main clause 8 in ISO 9001:2000 is thoroughly confusing to medical laboratory professionals who would immediately think of something done on the bench.

Main clauses of ISO 9001:2000	Clauses of the 'Ideal Standard'
1 Scope	1 Scope
2 Normative references	2 Source references
3 Terms and definitions	3 Terms and definitions
4 Quality management system	4 Quality management system
5 Management responsibility	5 Organization and management responsibility
6 Resource management	6 Resource management
7 Product realization	7 Examination processes
8 Measurement, analysis and improvement	8 Evaluation and continual improvement

Figure 3.4 The structure of ISO 9001:2000 and the 'Ideal Standard' compared

These changes in terminology then permit the creation of a model of a process-based quality management system for the medical laboratory (Figure 3.5) which, whilst retaining the essential features of the ISO 9001:2000 model, should be more familiar to medical laboratory professionals.

RELATIONSHIP BETWEEN THE PROCESS-BASED MODEL AND ISO 17025:1999

The relationship between the main clauses of process-based model (ISO 9001:2000/the 'Ideal Standard') and ISO 17025:1999 is shown in Figure 3.6. Two main clauses of ISO 17025:1999 (5.4 and 5.9) appear more than once because their content is applicable in more than one place. If more than one entry is made, the first one is shown for example as: 5.9 Assuring the quality of test and calibration results (1) etc. The main clause, 5.1 General, does not appear because it only serves to introduce other clauses.

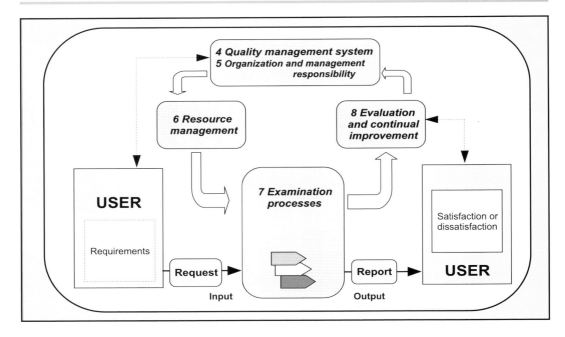

Figure 3.5 A process-based quality management system for the medical laboratory

If one wishes to use clauses of ISO 17025:1999 in the context of a process-based quality management scheme they can be placed in the appropriate boxes of Figures 3.5 and the standard used in the context of a medical laboratory. This should allow the introduction of ISO 17025:1999 in a manner that is of practical value to the laboratory and facilitates the training and education of all members of laboratory staff. The informative Annex B of ISO 17025:1999 provides 'Guidelines for establishing applications for specific fields'. This has been achieved in Hungary by a group of medical laboratory professionals working closely with the National Accreditation Board, Nemzeti Akkreditáló Testület.

RELATIONSHIP BETWEEN THE PROCESS-BASED MODEL AND ISO 15189:2002

A relationship between the main clauses of the process-based model (ISO:9001:2000/'Ideal Standard') and ISO 15189:2002 can be constructed in a similar manner and the information enabling this to be done can be found in Figure 2.12.

ISO 9001:2000 (term in the 'Ideal Standard')	ISO 17025:1999
4 Quality management system (Quality management system)	4.1 Organization 4.2 Quality system 4.3 Document control
5 Management responsibility (Organization and management responsibility)	4.4 Review of requests, tenders and contracts 4.12 Control of records 4.14 Management reviews
6 Resource management (Resource management)	4.6 Purchasing services and supplies 5.2 Personnel 5.3 Accomodation and environmental conditions 5.5 Equipment
7 Product realization (Examination processes)	4.5 Sub-contracting of tests and calibrations 4.7 Service to the client 5.7 Sampling 5.8 Handling of test and calibration items 5.4 Test and calibration methods and *method validation* (1) 5.4 *Test and calibration methods* and method validation (2) 5.6 Measurement traceability 5.9 Assuring the quality of test and calibration results (1) 5.10 Reporting results
8 Measurement, analysis improvement (Evaluation and continual improvement)	4.8 Complaints 4.9 Control of nonconforming testing and/or calibration work 4.10 Corrective action 4.11 Preventative action 4.13 Internal audits 5.9 Assuring the quality of test and calibration results (2)

Figure 3.6 Relationship between ISO 9001:2000/the 'Ideal Standard' and ISO 17025:1999

THE 'IDEAL STANDARD'

Figure 3.7 gives a sample of the structure of the 'Ideal Standard' and Appendix 1 provides a table of the complete structure, to second sub-clause level, of the provisions of an 'Ideal Standard' and cross references it to the following standards ISO 9001:2000, ISO 17025:1999, ISO 15189:2002 and CPA(UK) Ltd.

---

4   QUALITY MANAGEMENT SYSTEM
4.1   General requirements
4.2   Documentation requirements
      4.2.1   General
      4.2.2   Quality manual
      4.2.3   Control of documents
      4.2.4   Control of records
      4.2.5   Control of clinical material

5   ORGANIZATION AND MANAGEMENT RESPONSIBILITY
5.1   General management
5.2   Organization
5.3   Management responsibility
      5.3.1   Management commitment
      5.3.2   Needs and requirements of the users
      5.3.3   Quality policy
      5.3.4   Quality objectives and plans
      5.3.5   Responsibility, authority and communication
      5.3.6   Quality manager
      5.3.7   Management review

Figure 3.7 A sample of the structure of the 'Ideal Standard'

The structure was created using material from the headings of ISO 9001:2000, ISO 17025:1999, ISO 15189:2002, EC4 Essential Criteria and the current standards of CPA(UK)Ltd.

IT IS RECOMMENDED THAT THE READER MAKES A PHOTOCOPY OF APPENDIX 1 TO HAVE IT AVAILABLE AS A ROAD MAP TO ASSIST IN READING THE REST OF THIS BOOK.

BUILDING A QUALITY MANAGEMENT SYSTEM

In defining a *'management system'* as a 'system to establish policies and objectives and to achieve those objectives', ISO 9000:2000 'Quality management system – Fundamentals and vocabulary' draws attention to the fact that the overall management system of an organization can include different management systems, for example, systems for quality, environmental or financial manage-ment. Thus it defines a *'quality management system'* as a 'management system to direct and control an organization with regard to quality'. This section discusses the steps to be taken to establish, control, review and improve a quality manage-ment system (QMS).

The NPAAC has published a valuable document 'Guidelines for quality systems in medical laboratories'. Figure 3.8 is adapted from the quality system flowchart illustrated in the document and shows a structured approach to establishment, control, review and improvement of a quality management system.

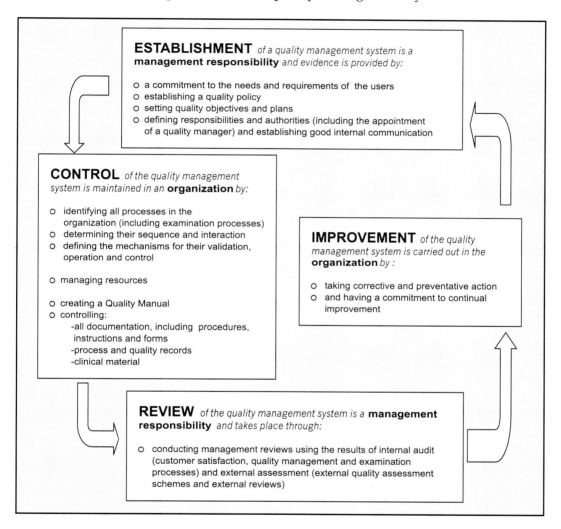

ESTABLISHMENT *of a quality management system is a* **management responsibility** *and evidence is provided by:*

o a commitment to the needs and requirements of the users
o establishing a quality policy
o setting quality objectives and plans
o defining responsibilities and authorities (including the appointment of a quality manager) and establishing good internal communication

CONTROL *of the quality management system is maintained in an* **organization** *by:*

o identifying all processes in the organization (including examination processes)
o determining their sequence and interaction
o defining the mechanisms for their validation, operation and control

o managing resources

o creating a Quality Manual
o controlling:
    -all documentation, including procedures, instructions and forms
    -process and quality records
    -clinical material

IMPROVEMENT *of the quality management system is carried out in the* **organization** *by :*

o taking corrective and preventative action
o and having a commitment to continual improvement

REVIEW *of the quality management system is a* **management responsibility** *and takes place through:*

o conducting management reviews using the results of internal audit (customer satisfaction, quality management and examination processes) and external assessment (external quality assessment schemes and external reviews)

Figure 3.8 Building a quality management system

Although the NPAAC document is primarily a practical guide to ISO 17025:1999 it is equally applicable to ISO 9001:2000 and ISO 15189:2002. The figure shows the four elements of the QMS; establishment, control, review and improvement, as a cycle. In each element a distinction is drawn between 'management responsibility', that focuses on the establishment and review elements, and an organization's responsibilities that focus on the control and improvement elements. In Chapter 4, management responsibility is described as being vested in 'laboratory management', the equivalent term in ISO 9001:2000 being 'top management'. This responsibility is executive in character, in contrast to the responsibility of an 'organization', which is corporate.

In Figure 3.4, the main clauses of an 'Ideal Standard' were presented along with their equivalents in ISO 9001:2000, and this figure is expanded below (Figure 3.9) to include the correlation with the elements of establishment, control, review and improvement of a QMS (Figure 3.8).

Main clauses of ISO 9001:2000	Clauses of the 'Ideal Standard'	Relationship to elements of a QMS (Figure 3.8)
1 Scope	1 Scope	*Not applicable*
2 Normative references	2 Source references	*Not applicable*
3 Terms and definitions	3 Terms and definitions	*Not applicable*
4 Quality management system	4 Quality management system	CONTROL
5 Management responsibility	5 Management responsibility	ESTABLISHMENT & REVIEW
6 Resource management	6 Resource management	CONTROL
7 Product realization	7 Examination processes	CONTROL
8 Measurement, analysis and improvement	8 Evaluation and continual improvement	IMPROVEMENT

Figure 3.9 Elements of a QMS in relation to ISO 9001:2000 and the 'Ideal Standard'

THE SEQUENCE OF ACTION IN QUALITY MANAGEMENT
As we have seen within the establishment and control stages of creating a QMS there is a sequence of action which is illustrated in Figure 3.10.

The first step in the sequence is *policies* which can be defined as the 'overall intentions and direction of an organization'. The second step *objectives and plans*, involves 'making plans and setting objectives to enable the fulfilment of the intentions expressed in the policies'. The third step *processes*, involves the 'definition of the activities needed to carry out the intentions' and the fourth step *procedures*, are the 'practical way in which intentions are translated into action'. The fifth and final step, *records* provide evidence, on a day to day basis, that procedures have been carried out correctly and that intentions have been fulfilled.

In terms of a medical laboratory this sequence would translate as follows. The quality policy of the laboratory includes a commitment to the reporting of results of examinations in a timely manner. The supplier of the laboratory computer system announces the release of a module for ward reporting of results. Laboratory management establishes the installation of this module as an objective for the next financial year. Planning for this development requires the inclusion of the resource implications in the business plan. Its impact on post-examination processes is defined and procedures reviewed and revised.

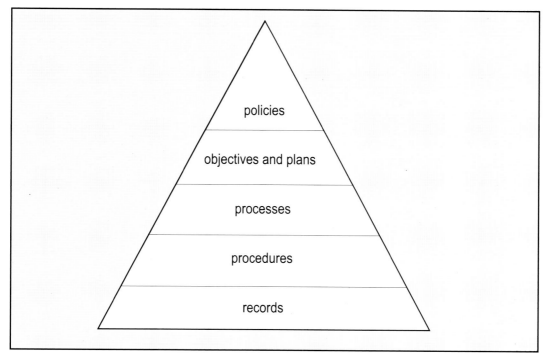

Figure 3.10 The sequence of action in quality management

An examination of the role of laboratory management in the establishment of a QMS is presented in Chapter 4, Organization and management responsibility. The control in terms of documentation in Chapter 5, in terms of management of resources in Chapters 6-8 and in terms of processes in Chapters 9 and 10 and review and improvement in Chapter 11.

Chapter 4

Organization and management responsibility

INTRODUCTION

'Ideal Standard' clause 5 Organization and management responsibility

In Chapter 3 the reader was introduced to the 'Ideal Standard' for medical laboratories and in this chapter an 'ideal laboratory' makes its appearance. This laboratory started life in the author's first book 'Understanding Accreditation in Laboratory Medicine' as the Pathology Laboratory in the Clinical Directorate of Diagnostic and Therapeutic Services of St Elsewhere's Hospital Trust. In its renaissance, it continues to consist of departments of Biochemistry, Haematology, Microbiology and Histopathology, but is in the process of becoming part of a larger co-operation of pathology services serving a population of 1.3 million people. It is hoped as these chapters unfold, that the pathology laboratory of St Elsewhere's will become a virtual reality.

This chapter concerns the management of a laboratory, (organization and management responsibility) and relates to the requirements of main clause 5 of the 'Ideal Standard'. The inter-connectivity of these requirements is illustrated in Figure 4.1, which is intended to provide both a process-based diagram and a route map to the chapter.

The chapter is presented in four main sections. The first section of the chapter presents an outline structure of a procedure for management of the laboratory. The second deals not with *'organization'*, as defined in ISO 9001:2000 as 'a group of people and facilities with an arrangement of responsibilities, authorities and relationships' (in ISO 17025:1999 and ISO 15189:2002, the equivalent term would be *'laboratory'*), but rather with the attributes or characteristics of a laboratory that contribute to its ability to demonstrate competence.

In the third section, *'organization'* is dealt with as an arrangement of responsibilities, authorities and relationships and forms one of the aspects of *'management responsibility'*. In the final section the purpose, preparation and content of a quality manual is introduced. At the end of the chapter pages from the Quality Manual of the Pathology Laboratory illustrate the approach to the organization and management responsibility in St Elsewhere's Hospital Trust.

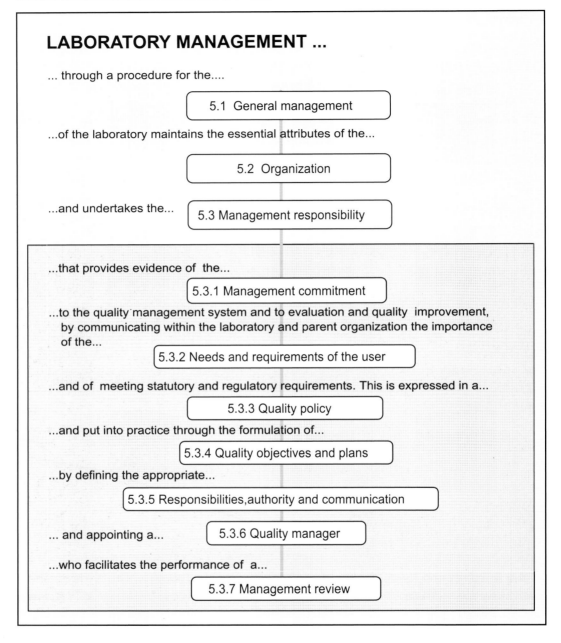

LABORATORY MANAGEMENT ...

... through a procedure for the....

5.1 General management

...of the laboratory maintains the essential attributes of the...

5.2 Organization

...and undertakes the...

5.3 Management responsibility

...that provides evidence of the...

5.3.1 Management commitment

...to the quality management system and to evaluation and quality improvement, by communicating within the laboratory and parent organization the importance of the...

5.3.2 Needs and requirements of the user

...and of meeting statutory and regulatory requirements. This is expressed in a...

5.3.3 Quality policy

...and put into practice through the formulation of...

5.3.4 Quality objectives and plans

...by defining the appropriate...

5.3.5 Responsibilities,authority and communication

... and appointing a...

5.3.6 Quality manager

...who facilitates the performance of a...

5.3.7 Management review

Figure 4.1 Main clause 5 of the 'Ideal Standard' – Organization and management responsibility

GENERAL MANAGEMENT
'Ideal Standard' clause 5.1 General management

The contents page of the procedure for general management of the pathology laboratory [MP-GEN-PathMan]* is shown in Figure 4.2. At St Elsewhere's the relationships between the laboratory and the Trust, and within pathology are illustrated in the overview of the organization section of the Quality Manual [QM-GEN-QualMan] (see Figures 4.15 and 4.16). The Director of Pathology, is responsible for implementation of general management procedure and the main evidence of its functioning would be the minutes of meetings (see Figure 5.19) of the Pathology Management Board, its sub-committees and working groups.

The frequency of meetings of the Board and its sub-committees should be defined and will depend on how much of the day to day management is conducted at the Board or delegated to sub-committees or working groups. The balance between what should be dealt with by the Board and what should be dealt with by sub-committees or working groups is a difficult one. The Board should perhaps be more concerned with strategic rather than operational matters, and membership of sub-committees should be seen as an opportunity for a broader group of staff to participate in the management of pathology. For example, at St Elsewhere's the annual management review is discussed and agreed by a full meeting of the Board, but the preparatory work is done by the Quality and Accreditation Committee. The Board should meet at least once a month if it is going to maintain continuity and effectively communicate its decisions.

The agenda of the Board meetings should have an agreed structure which would include reports from sub-committees and working groups on a regular basis. The minutes should record decisions taken, and where further action is required, it should carefully define the responsibility for reporting back and the time limit. Minutes of the Board and its sub-committees are evidence that procedure for general management is working satisfactorily. They should indicate that the Board is able not only to make decisions, but also to implement them within the resources available.

---

* Further detail of 'informative filenames' is to be found in Chapter 5 Documentation

St Elsewhere's Hospital Trust	Edition: 1.0	Filename: MP-GEN-PathMan
	Author: J. Qualiman	Authorized by: W.Jaggard
PATHOLOGY LABORATORY	Date of issue: 05/01/2001	Page: 2/12

TABLE OF CONTENTS

Figure 4.2 Contents page of the procedure for the management of pathology [MP-GEN-PathMan]

ORGANIZATION

'Ideal Standard' clause 5.2 Organization

The 'Management requirements' clauses of both ISO 17025:1999 and ISO 15189:2002 have a section on organization and/or management. Most of this section of the chapter relates to the responsibilities of management (management responsibility), but a part concerns the attributes or characteristics of a laboratory that contribute to its ability to demonstrate competence, particularly in terms of its ethical behaviour (Figure 4.3). Ethical behaviour is defined as behaviour that is 'in accordance with principles of conduct which are considered correct'. The perception of what is correct conduct will undergo change with time as has been graphically demonstrated by recent responses to the problems of consent and the retention of organs by medical laboratories in the UK. That such perception changes is illustrated by an interesting and important requirement in the recent 'Draft Standards for Pathology Laboratories' published in Australia by the NPAAC and shown in italics in Figure 4.3. This requirement to 'have policies and procedures to ensure there are acceptable standards of staff conduct towards human samples, tissues or remains' is taken from Standard 3, Laboratory Ethics, and is not clearly expressed in ISO standards.

A laboratory should...

- be an entity that can be held legally responsible

- have arrangements that ensure that all personnel are free from undue internal and external pressures and influences that may adversely affect their work

- have arrangements that avoid involvement in any activities that would diminish confidence in its impartiality, judgement and operational integrity

- have arrangements that protect user's confidential information

- *have policies and procedures to ensure there are acceptable standards of staff conduct towards human samples, tissues or remains (NPACC)*

- meet the requirements of the Standard to satisfy the needs of users, regulatory bodies or bodies providing recognition (e.g. an accreditation body)

Figure 4.3 Attributes or characteristics of a laboratory

At St Elsewhere's the Quality Policy (Figure 4.6) states that the laboratory will 'uphold professional values and be committed to good professional practice and conduct' and details its approach in its Quality Manual.

LEGAL ENTITY

In ISO 15189:2002 there is a requirement for the laboratory to be a 'legal entity'. It is not entirely clear what this means until the equivalent clauses of ISO 17025:1999 and ISO/IEC DIS 17011 are examined. These indicate that the laboratory itself, or the organization of which it is a part, 'shall be an entity that can be held legally responsible for all its activities'. A note is added to the effect that laboratories that are publicly funded or part of government will be deemed to be legal entities. In different countries the nature of being a legal entity will be determined by national legislation, but in practical terms, this means being an entity that is contactable by virtue of having premises with facilities for communication by post, telephone, fax or email. At St Elsewhere's this information is provided in the General Information section of the Quality Manual (see Figure 4.13).

GENERAL ATTRIBUTES

The remaining attributes of a laboratory that contribute to its competence require evidence not only that the laboratory itself has in place necessary mechanisms, but that the individuals who work for the organization understand, accept and comply with the need for these mechanisms (Figure 4.4). The practical ways in which these arrangements are discharged are discussed in Chapter 6 under personnel management and in Chapters 9 and 10 on examination processes.

MANAGEMENT RESPONSIBILITY
'Ideal Standard' clause 5.3 Management responsibility
In the terms and definitions section of ISO 9000:2000, *'management'* is defined as 'co-ordinated activities to direct and control an organization', but a note suggests that if the word is to be used in the sense of 'the members of the executive or administration of an organization' it should be preceded by a qualifier. For example in ISO 9001:2000 the term *'top management'* is used whereas in ISO 17025:1999 and ISO 15189:2002 the equivalent term is *'laboratory management'*.

In ISO 9001:2000, the terms, *'top management'* and *'organization'* are used with great precision and the use of the phrase 'top management shall…' is confined to the requirements detailed in main clause 5, 'Management responsibility and organization'. In all other sections of the standard the phrase, 'the organization shall…' is used for requirements that require corporate rather than executive responsibility.

ATTRIBUTES	EVIDENCE Internal action	External action
1 Personnel free from undue internal and external pressures and influences that may adversely affect their work	Voluntary register of potential conflicts of interest such as other remunerated and unremunerated work Sickness and overtime records	Compliance with national employment and health provision legislation
2 Avoidance of involvement in any activities that would diminish confidence in its impartiality, judgement and operational integrity	Compliance with a code of conduct regarding acceptance of gifts from third parties	Membership of statutory or voluntary register Membership of a professional body with a written code of conduct
3 Arrangements that protect the user's confidential information	Item in laboratory induction programme Controlled access to the laboratory Security system for computer access	Registration in conformity with national legislation on data protection
4 Have policies and procedures to ensure there are acceptable standards of staff conduct towards human samples, tissues or remains	Procedures for consent, collection, transportation, storage of human samples, tissues or remains	
5 Meet the requirements of the Standards to satisfy the needs of users and regulatory or accreditation bodies	Certificates from external organizations Paragraph in job description requiring compliance with Standards	Reports from external agencies, Health & Safety, Radiological Protection etc.

Figure 4.4 Evidence of compliance with attributes or characteristics of a laboratory

The terms equivalent to top management and organization are 'laboratory management' and 'laboratory', but in ISO 17025:1999 and ISO 15189:2002 they are used with much less precision. Thus ISO 17025:1999, states 'The laboratory shall establish, implement and maintain a quality system…', whereas ISO 15189:2002, states 'The laboratory management shall have responsibility for the design, implementation, maintenance, and improvement of the quality management system…'. To compound the lack of clarity, the sub-clause on management review in ISO 17025:1999 uses the phrase 'the laboratory's executive management shall…', implying an extra tier of management in addition to laboratory management. In this book, *'laboratory management'* is seen as 'those persons who direct and control the laboratory at the top level'. This approach is in keeping with the ISO 9001:2000 concept of top management and puts the focus on the management responsibilities to be discharged in relation to the provision of a service to users, rather than the qualifications or competencies required for the role of laboratory director, which may be best determined by local circumstances and legislation.

However, the standards in some accreditation systems require that Laboratory Directors/Heads of Department should have defined competencies and be appropriately qualified to take overall responsibility. This special aspect of laboratory management is discussed further in Chapter 6. The prime responsibilities of management described in this section are a re-echo of the responsibilities of laboratory management in establishing and reviewing the quality management system (Figure 3.8) and the relationships of these responsibilities that are shown graphically in Figure 4.1.

MANAGEMENT COMMITMENT
'Ideal Standard' clause 5.3.1 Management commitment
The concept of leadership is expounded as one of the principles of quality management (see Figure 3.3) in ISO 9000:2000. Leadership is seen as establishing a unity of purpose in an organization (laboratory), providing a direction and creating an environment in which all personnel can contribute.

NEEDS AND REQUIREMENTS OF THE USERS
'Ideal Standard' clause 5.3.2 Needs and requirements of users
The *'user'* of the laboratory is generally considered to be the clinician who makes a request on behalf of a patient in their charge. Less commonly the patient is a direct user, for example if the laboratory is involved in training a patient to use a glucose monitoring device. This type of involvement is exemplified in the description of a medical laboratory service (Figure 3.1) as including the potential for a presence 'in the home'. A third use of the term 'user' is when a third party, for example, a healthcare organization is purchasing services from a laboratory. It is important that such contractual arrangements involve the laboratory in direct relationships with the referring clinician. A medical laboratory is not a factory for examination (analytical) processes. The needs and requirements of the users should be formulated in a Users Manual (Chapter 9, Pre- and post-examination processes) and continually monitored and evaluated (Chapter 11, Evaluation and quality improvement).

QUALITY POLICY
'Ideal Standard' clause 5.3.3 Quality policy
ISO 9000:2000 defines a quality policy as the 'overall intentions and direction of

an organization related to quality as formally expressed by management'. In effect it represents a public commitment to the needs and requirements of the user. Only ISO 17025:1999 gives any detail as to the possible content of a quality policy, although other ISO standards require that (laboratory) management include a commitment to comply with the requirements of the standards. Laboratory management should also ensure its appropriateness, make sure it is communicated and understood within the laboratory and that it is reviewed on a regular basis. It is important that it is seen as policy that concerns not just quality but all aspects of the management of quality in the laboratory, from producing quality results through to the safe disposal of waste. The requirements in ISO 17025:1999 for the content of a quality policy are summarised in Figure 4.5.

A quality policy should include...

- a commitment to good professional practice and to the provision of quality testing (examinations)

- a statement of the laboratory's standards of service

- a description of the objectives of the quality system

- a requirement that all personnel familiarise themselves with the documentation and implement the policies and procedures in their work

- a commitment by laboratory management to compliance with the standard upon which the laboratory operates

---

Figure 4.5 Content of a quality policy

This theoretical content is translated into 'The Quality Policy of the Pathology laboratory of St Elsewhere's Hospital Trust' [MF-GEN-QualPol] in Figure 4.6. This is based upon a template developed by CPA(UK)Ltd.

QUALITY OBJECTIVES AND PLANS
'Ideal Standard' clause 5.3.4 Quality objectives and plans
Whereas the quality policy should be regularly reviewed, it is unlikely that it will be subject to frequent change. In contrast, quality objectives and plans will need revision on a regular basis as they are the means through which the commitments made in the Quality Policy are delivered and maintained. Measurable objectives that are consistent with the maintenance of the quality policy need to be set for relevant functions and levels within the laboratory. These objectives, and the plans which are prepared to carry these objectives through, will need regular review as to their effectiveness. As ISO 9001:2000 clearly relates quality objectives

and plans to the quality management system (QMS), it is important to underline that the QMS or management of quality includes all activities in the laboratory.

THE QUALITY POLICY OF THE PATHOLOGY LABORATORY OF ST ELSEWHERE'S HOSPITAL TRUST

The Pathology Laboratory is committed to providing a service of the highest quality and shall be aware and take into consideration the needs and requirements of its users.

In order to ensure that the needs and requirements of users are met, the Pathology Laboratory will:

- operate a quality management system to integrate the organization, procedures, processes and resources
- set quality objectives and plans in order to implement and maintain this quality policy
- ensure that all personnel are familiar with this quality policy to ensure user satisfaction
- commit to the health, safety and welfare of all its staff
- ensure that visitors to the department will be treated with respect and that due consideration will be given to their safety while on site
- uphold professional values and be committed to good professional practice and conduct

The Pathology Laboratory will comply with standards set by the 'Ideal Standard' and is committed to:

- staff recruitment, training, development and retention at all levels to provide a full and effective service to its users
- the proper procurement and maintenance of such equipment and other resources as are needed for the provision of the service
- the collection, transport and handling of all specimens in such a way as to ensure the correct performance of laboratory examinations
- the use of examination procedures that will ensure the highest achievable quality of all tests performed
- reporting results of examinations in ways which are timely, confidential, accurate and clinically useful
- the assessment of user satisfaction, in addition to internal audit and external quality assessment, in order to produce continual quality improvement.

SIGNED ON BEHALF OF THE PATHOLOGY LABORATORY

Director of Pathology   William   Jaggard   **Date** 2 January 2001

MF-GEN-QualPol

Based on a template provided by CPA(UK)Ltd

Figure 4.6 Quality Policy of the laboratory of St Elsewhere's Hospital Trust

An example of how quality policy, objectives, and plans interact is as follows. The laboratory at St Elsewhere's has made a policy commitment to 'reporting results of examinations in ways which are timely, confidential, accurate and clinically useful'. In the development of co-operation between itself and two other similar laboratories, a prime objective is to unify the laboratory computer systems and their reporting links with the patient management systems (PMS). At the two other hospitals the laboratory system has no links with PMS and very careful planning will be required to meet the objective whilst still retaining the policy commitment.

RESPONSIBILITY, AUTHORITY AND COMMUNICATION
'Ideal Standard' clause 5.3.5 Responsibility, authority and communication
Successful implementation of standards does not depend so much on how different laboratories are organized, or what the Head of Department is called, but on a clear definition of its organization, its attributes and the responsibilities of laboratory management. The importance of the Quality Manual in encompassing this information is discussed later in the chapter and its role as an index or road map to the documentation of the laboratory leads into Chapter 5.

There are many different ways in which a pathology laboratory can be organized. In large hospitals, particularly large teaching hospital laboratories, the pathology disciplines tend to operate as fully or semi-autonomous departments. In the medium sized district general hospital like St Elsewhere's, the pathology laboratory is composed of a group of individual disciplines or departments. In small hospitals or their equivalent, the laboratory is often a single multidisciplinary entity with no separate departments. In both the public and private sectors there is an increasing trend to co-operations between already large units of pathology provision creating a significant imperative for effective management arrangements and proper control of documentation (see Chapter 5).

The functioning and effectiveness of a pathology laboratory can be hindered or enhanced by the quality of its relationship with its parent body or host organization. In most cases this will be a hospital, but in some cases it will be a holding company, and management of the laboratory will be independent of any of the hospitals which it serves. This relationship is a management relationship outside the laboratory (Figure 4.15). Equal in importance, is how the organizational structure and management within the laboratory (Figure 4.16) impacts upon the way it functions. It will affect not only the quality of the results, but also have a marked effect on the staff who work in the laboratory. Organizations must be structured to meet local needs, and some fundamental principles suggested in a report of the Audit Commission (UK) are shown in Figure 4.7.

A management structure should have...

- clear demarcation of responsibilities

- clear reporting lines

- well established and well used lines of communication

- functions discharged at an appropriate level

'The Pathology Services: A Management Review' Audit Commission (1991)

Figure 4.7 Fundamental principles for organization and management

If an organization (laboratory) is to be regarded as 'a group of people and facilities with an arrangement of responsibilities, authorities and relationships', these concepts need to be represented in an easily understood and well defined manner. One way of doing this is to use organization charts or as they are sometimes called 'organograms'. In creating such charts it is important to be clear what is to be represented. For example, is it the relationship between facilities that is to be represented, or the relationships and authorities between people, or both?

Although it is often said that 'a diagram is worth a thousand words', creating meaningful organizational charts is notoriously difficult and sometimes words may be better. In St Elsewhere's Hospital Trust, the reader can choose between a description of the current situation as 'the pathology laboratory is part of the Directorate of Diagnostic and Therapeutic Medicine and comprises the Departments of Biochemistry, Haematology, Microbiology and Histopathology and is managed by the Pathology Management Board' and/or as organizational charts shown in the opening pages of the Quality Manual illustrated in Figures 4.15 and 4.16. For further use of organization charts in job descriptions see Figure 6.7 in Chapter 6.

QUALITY MANAGER
'Ideal Standard' clause 5.3.6 Quality manager
ISO 9001:2000, ISO 17025:1999 and ISO 15189:2002 all require the appointment of a *'quality manager'* (however named). In ISO 9001:2000 this post is called the 'management representative' which provides the first clue as to the nature of this very important appointment. ISO 17025:1999 requires that 'irrespective of other duties and responsibilities...' the quality manager shall have 'defined responsibility and authority for ensuring that the quality system is implemented and followed at all times...' and have 'direct access to the highest level of management

at which decisions are made on laboratory policy or resources'. The CPA standard A7 Quality manager, is illustrated in Figure 4.8 and attempts to incorporate all the key requirements into the practical setting of a medical laboratory. In particular it is important to see the role as ensuring that the QMS is implemented and maintained, as distinct from undertaking all the tasks, for example, scheduling internal audits rather than necessarily performing them. The role for a quality manager is discussed further in Chapter 11.

A7 Quality manager
The quality manager is the individual who ensures, on behalf of laboratory management, that the quality management system functions correctly

A7.1 Laboratory management or management of the parent organization shall appoint a quality manager [NOTE 1].

A7.2 The quality manager's reporting arrangements shall be agreed between laboratory management and management of the parent organization.

A7.3 The quality manager, irrespective of other responsibilities [NOTE 2], shall have defined authority for:

a) ensuring the quality management system is implemented and maintained

b) reporting to laboratory management on the functioning and effectiveness of the quality management system

c) co-ordinating awareness of the needs and requirements of users.

NOTES
1. The quality manager should have responsibility for the implementation and maintenance of the quality management system, but not for undertaking all the tasks involved. The term quality manager is comparable with management representative (as described in ISO 9001:2000 para 5.5.5)
2. The quality manager may be engaged full time or part time on quality management and may or may not have other responsibilities in the parent organization or the laboratory.

CPA (UK) Ltd Standards for the Medical Laboratory 2001

Figure 4.8 CPA(UK)Ltd Standard A7 Quality manager

MANAGEMENT REVIEW
'Ideal Standard' clause 5.3.7 Management review
The requirement for a *'management review'* is clearly expressed in ISO 9001:2000, ISO 17025:1999 and ISO 15189:2002. The description of a management review and practical ways in which it can be implemented will be described in Chapter 11.

QUALITY MANUAL
'Ideal Standard' clause 4.2.2 Quality manual
With only a few exceptions, the standards which underpin accreditation systems

throughout the world require a quality manual. This section looks at the purpose of a quality manual, introduces a possible structure and content and provides as an illustration, the opening pages of the Quality Manual of the Pathology Laboratory of St Elsewhere's Hospital Trust which is based on the requirements of the 'Ideal Standard'. There are a number of texts which give information on the format and content of a quality manual, including ISO 10013:1995(E) 'Guidelines for developing quality manuals' (Figure 4.9). The illustrative material provided incorporates those guidelines.

---

1. Title, scope and field of application.

2. Table of contents.

3. Introductory pages about the organization concerned and the manual itself.

4. Quality policy and objectives of the organization.

5. Description of the organization, structure, responsibilities and authorities.

6. Description of the elements of the quality system and any references to documented quality system procedures.

7. Definitions section, if appopriate.

8. Index to the quality manual.

9. Appendix for supportive data.

based on ISO 10013:1995 Guidelines for developing quality manuals

---

Figure 4.9 Content of a quality manual

PURPOSE OF A QUALITY MANUAL

A quality manual is a useful document in relation to a number of different groups of people (Figure 4.10). It provides information which should dovetail with the management activities of the host organization. Laboratory management has the prime responsibility for establishing and reviewing the quality management system and the quality manual and the quality policy reinforce the commitments made by laboratory management.

The quality manual enables laboratory personnel to understand management's commitment to quality and, when the time comes for outside assessors to visit the laboratory to assess compliance with the accreditation standards, the quality manual forms a starting point for the assessment. Finally, it can be given to users to assure them of a commitment to quality. In this last sense it can be used in marketing to attract new custom. With these different uses in mind it is important that the quality manual should be up to date, clearly and succinctly written, and attractively produced.

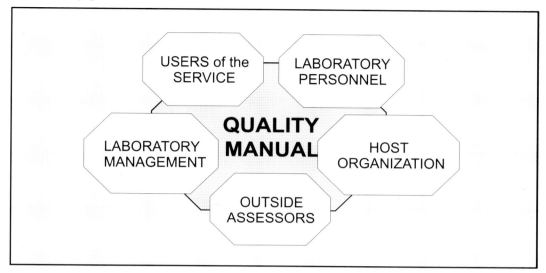

Figure 4.10   Purposes of a quality manual

PREPARATION AND CONTROL OF THE QUALITY MANUAL
At St Elsewhere's once the management decision had been made to document the quality or accreditation system in a quality manual, the job was delegated to the Quality Manager. The Quality Manager worked with the Quality and Accreditation Committee, to co-ordinate the production, subsequent review and revision of the manual. A recommended maximum length is twenty five pages. The process of document control described in Chapter 5 applies to the quality manual. Any copies issued outside the pathology laboratory for purposes of information to present or potential users should be clearly marked as uncon-trolled copies.

CONTENT OF THE QUALITY MANUAL
The content of a quality manual as suggested in ISO 10013:1995 was shown in Figure 4.9. The opening pages of a quality manual are discussed in the following paragraphs and are illustrated in Figures 4.11-4.16 which show the opening pages of the Quality Manual for the pathology laboratory of St Elsewhere's. Other sources of information for the structure and content of quality manuals are provided in Appendix 2 Further Reading.

TITLE, SCOPE AND FIELD OF APPLICATION

The front page or the cover (Figure 4.11) gives the title, and in the case of the Quality Manual, its scope and field of application. Document identification and control information is given in the page header, (see Chapter 5 for further information). In countries where accreditation is still voluntary, a particular department in Pathology might decide not to apply for accreditation. If this is the case then this should be stated clearly on the title page.

TABLE OF CONTENTS

The table of contents should contain the title of the main sections, and the numbering of the sections should be shown, together with the page number. If the quality manual is based directly upon a particular standard, then it is very helpful if the numbering of the contents follows the numbering in the standard. In the case of the laboratory at St Elsewhere's which follows the 'Ideal Standard', the contents page (Figure 4.12) and the headings of the 'Ideal Standard' in Appendix 1 indicate how this can be achieved.

GENERAL INFORMATION

The introductory page of the quality manual should provide basic information about the laboratory and provide evidence that the laboratory has a 'legal identity' (Figure 4.13).

QUALITY POLICY

After the introductory pages there follows the laboratory's quality policy (Figure 4.14). The function and purpose of a Quality Policy has been discussed earlier in the chapter and it can be reproduced as a stand alone document [MF-GEN-QualPol].

DEFINITIONS

This section includes terms used in a technical sense in the manual and their definitions. This page of the quality manual is not illustrated.

OVERVIEW OF THE ORGANIZATION, RESPONSIBILITIES AND AUTHORITIES

This section contains information concerning the relationship between the pathology laboratory and the parent body or host organization (Figure 4.15). If the quality manual is written for an individual pathology discipline, then the relationship of that department to the pathology laboratory and the host organization should be included. The organization, responsibilities and authorities within the laboratory are presented as a brief diagrammatic overview (Figure 4.16). In the case of the laboratory at St Elsewhere's, the further detail of these is contained in the procedure for the management of the pathology laboratory (Figure 4.2).

RESPONSE TO THE REQUIREMENTS OF THE STANDARD

The major section of the quality manual (in the case of the laboratory at St Elsewhere's, on pages 8-24) contains clear statements of how the laboratory complies with the requirements of the 'Ideal Standard' and references appropriate procedures. An example of this is shown for the QMS including documentation requirements in Figure 5.4.

St Elsewhere's Hospital Trust	**Edition:** 1.0	**Filename:** QM-GEN-QualMan
	Author: J. Qualiman	**Authorized by:** W. Jaggard
PATHOLOGY LABORATORY	**Date of issue:** 03/01/2001	Page 1/24

QUALITY MANUAL

- This document, together with procedures specified in this manual, represent the quality management system of the Pathology Laboratory of St Elsewhere's Hospital Trust.
- It has been compiled to meet the requirements of the 'Ideal Standard' Accreditation System and appropriate national and international standards.
- All procedures specified herein are mandatory within the Pathology Laboratory

COPY	1/3
LOCATION OF COPIES	1. Office - Director of Pathology
	2. Office - Quality Manager
	3. Pathology Laboratory

Document review history			
Review date	**Reviewed by**	**Signature**	**Date**
January 2002	John Qualiman	John Qualiman	2 January 2002
January 2003			
January 2004			
January 2005			

Figure 4.11 Quality manual – front page

St Elsewhere's Hospital Trust	**Edition:** 1.0	**Filename:** QM-GEN-QualMan
	Author: J. Qualiman	**Authorized by:** W. Jaggard
PATHOLOGY LABORATORY	**Date of issue:** 03/01/2001	**Page:** 2/24

TABLE OF CONTENTS

Figure 4.12 Quality manual – contents page

0 GENERAL INFORMATION

The Pathology Laboratory of St Elsewhere's Hospital Trust is situated in the main hospital building on Level 5 East Wing. It is composed of four departments, Biochemistry, Haematology, Microbiology and Histopathology, and is part of the Clinical Directorate of Diagnostic and Therapeutic Services.

St Elsewhere's Hospital Trust provides a wide range of services to the population of St Elsewhere and the surrounding district of East Loanshire. The resident population is approximately 560,000. In addition to the usual facilities of a District General Hospital there are two specialised units, a renal dialysis unit and a cardiac transplant unit, which serve the whole county of Loanshire.

The Pathology Laboratory provides services to the main hospital, to Thorbury Hospital for the severely mentally handicapped. Twice daily courier runs for collection of samples, and electronic transmission of results, enables the provision of effective pathology services for the 350 primary care physicians and their patients in East Loanshire. The Pathology Laboratory is also responsible for the provision of all near patient testing facilities in the main hospital.

The postal address is:-

> Pathology Laboratory,
>
> St Elsewhere's Hospital Trust,
>
> Eastside Street,
>
> ST ELSEWHERE   Telephone (0800) 100200
>
> East Loanshire,   FAX   (0800) 300400
>
> EL7 5XX   E-mail   enquiries@pathlab-stelsewhere.uk

Further information on the services provided, and telephone numbers, are provided in the USERS HANDBOOK, **[LP-GEN-UserHbk]** copies of which can be obtained from the Pathology Business Manager telephone 0800 00201

Figure 4.13 Quality manual – general information

St Elsewhere's Hospital Trust	**Edition:** 1.0	**Filename:** QM-GEN-QualMan
	Author: J. Qualiman	**Authorized by:** W. Jaggard
PATHOLOGY LABORATORY	**Date of issue:** 03/01/2001	**Page:** 4/24

1 QUALITY POLICY

The Quality Policy of the Pathology Laboratory is given below and is also published as a separate controlled document, **[MF-GEN-QualPol]** for display in public areas of the laboratory.

The Pathology Laboratory is committed to providing a service of the highest quality and shall be aware and take into consideration the needs and requirements of its users.

In order to ensure that the needs and requirements of users are met, the Pathology Laboratory will:

- operate a quality management system to integrate the organization, procedures, processes and resources

- set quality objectives and plans in order to implement this quality policy

- ensure that all personnel are familiar with this quality policy to ensure user satisfaction

- commit to the health, safety and welfare of all its staff

- ensure that visitors to the department will be treated with respect and due consideration will be given to their safety while on site

- uphold professional values and be committed to good professional practice and conduct.

The Pathology Laboratory will comply with standards set by the 'Ideal Standard' accreditation system and is committed to:

- staff recruitment, training, development and retention at all levels to provide a full and effective service to its users

- the proper procurement and maintenance of the equipment and other resources needed for the provision of the service

- the collection, transport and handling of all specimens in such a way as to ensure the correct performance of laboratory examinations

- the use of examination procedures that will ensure the highest achievable quality of all tests performed

- reporting results of examinations in ways which are timely, confidential, accurate and clinically useful

the assessment of user satisfaction, in addition to internal audit and external quality assessment, in order to produce continual quality improvement.

Figure 4.14 Quality manual – quality policy

St Elsewhere's Hospital Trust	Edition: 1.0	Filename: QM-GEN-QualMan
	Author: J. Qualiman	Authorized by: W. Jaggard
PATHOLOGY LABORATORY	Date of issue: 03/01/2001	Page: 6/24

3 OVERVIEW OF THE ORGANIZATION, RESPONSIBILITIES AND AUTHORITIES

3.1 RELATIONSHIP TO ST ELSEWHERE'S HOSPITAL TRUST

The Pathology Laboratory is part of the clinical Directorate of Diagnostic and Therapeutic Medicine. The organizational relationships of that Directorate within St Elsewhere's Hospital Trust are shown below:

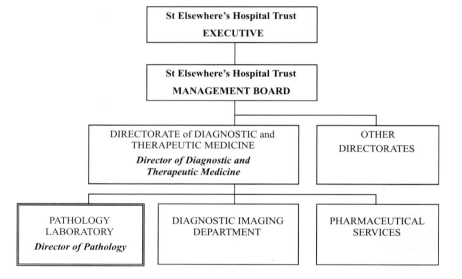

The *Director of Diagnostic and Therapeutic Medicine* is a member of the St Elsewhere's Management Board and is represented on the Executive by the Medical Director of the Trust.

The *Director of Pathology* is managerially responsible to the Director of Diagnostic and Therapeutic Medicine.

The *Director of Pathology* is the delegated Budget Holder for the Pathology Laboratory within the Directorate of Diagnostic and Therapeutic Medicine.

Figure 4.15   Quality manual – relationship of Pathology Laboratory to St Elsewhere's Hospital Trust

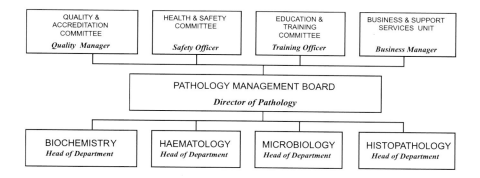

St Elsewhere's Hospital Trust | **Edition:** 1.0 | **Filename:** QM-GEN-QualMan
| **Author:** J. Qualiman | **Authorized by:** W. Jaggard
PATHOLOGY LABORATORY | **Date of issue:** 03/01/2001 | **Page:** 7/24

3.2 ORGANIZATION AND RESPONSIBILITIES WITHIN THE PATHOLOGY LABORATORY

The Pathology Laboratory has four main departments, each with a Head of Department and Chief Technologist. In departments with more than one Consultant Pathologist or Clinical Scientist, the headship is held on a rotating basis.

The membership of the Management Board of the Pathology Laboratory is as follows:-

- Director of Pathology (Chairperson)
- Heads of Departments
- Chief Technologist of each department
- Quality Manager
- Business Manager

The management of the Pathology Department is conducted using the procedure **[MP-GEN-PathMan]** and the proceedings recorded using **[MF-GEN-Minutes].** The Board is supported by a business and support services unit and three committees as shown above.

- The *Business Manager* is full time and responsible for Business, Computing and the Common Services (reception, secretarial and clerical services, for blood collection, for transport and purchasing).
- The *Training Officer* and a full time *Computer Manager* report to the *Business Manager*.
- The *Quality Manager* is full time and reports directly to the *Director of Pathology*
- The *Safety Officer* reports to the Board through the *Head of Microbiology*, attending as required

Figure 4.16 Quality manual – relationships within the pathology laboratory

Chapter 5

A quality management system and documentation

INTRODUCTION

'Ideal Standard' clause 4 Quality management system

In Chapter 3 the reader was introduced to the concepts of quality management for the medical laboratory. This chapter translates those concepts into the practical tools of a quality management system (QMS). Figure 5.1 illustrates the inter-connectivity of Main clause 4 of the 'Ideal Standard' which is concerned with the quality management system (QMS) and documentation requirements. It provides both a process based diagram and a route map to the chapter.

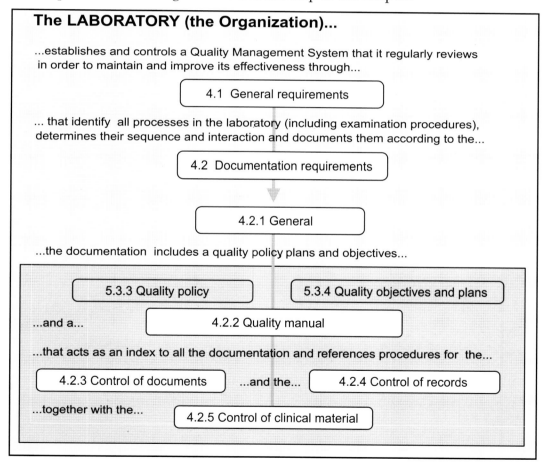

Figure 5.1 Main clause 4 of the 'Ideal Standard' – Quality management system

GENERAL REQUIREMENTS FOR A QUALITY MANAGEMENT SYSTEM

'Ideal Standard' clause 4.1 General requirements

In the last chapter the purpose, preparation and content of a Quality Manual [QM-GEN-QualMan] was discussed and illustrative opening pages of the quality manual from the laboratory of St Elsewhere's Hospital were presented (Figures 4.11-4.16).

Detailed requirements for creating an effective quality management system are set out in ISO 9001:2000 and Figure 5.2 is based on those requirements.

The laboratory shall...

- identify the processes required for the quality management system and their application throughout the laboratory

- determine the sequence and interaction of these processes

- ensure effective operation and control of these processes

- ensure that resource and information is available to support these processes

- continually evaluate these processes

- implement any actions required to maintain and improve the quality management system

based on ISO 9001:2000, clause 4.1 General requirements

Figure 5.2 General requirements of a quality management system

DOCUMENTATION REQUIREMENTS

'Ideal Standard' clause 4.2 Documentation requirements

GENERAL

'Ideal Standard' clause 4.2.1 General

The documentation requirements stem from the general requirements of a QMS and from the sequence of action in quality management described in Chapter 3 and illustrated in Figure 3.10. Figure 5.3 shows the hierachy of documentation which results from the implementation of this sequence of action.

At the top of this hierarchy is the *quality manual* that contains the *quality policy(s)*, and describes the processes that take place in the laboratory in order to fulfil the requirements of the standard with which the laboratory is seeking compliance.

Examples of such processes are, the procurement of equipment, the examination of specimens and the reporting of results. A policy can be defined as *'setting out the commitment of an organization to follow a particular course of action'*. A pathology laboratory can have a single policy statement which is inclusive of all aspects of its work or there can be a number of separate policies relating to different aspects of the laboratory's working. The quality policy itself will be subject to periodic review but is unlikely to change significantly unless the primary purpose of the laboratory were to change. However in order to pursue and maintain a particular course of action, *objectives* have to be set and *plans* executed. In contrast to the quality policy, objectives and plans are constantly changing in response to the changing needs and requirements of the users. The processes involved in this are set out in the Quality Manual, particularly in relation to the annual management review (Chapter 11).

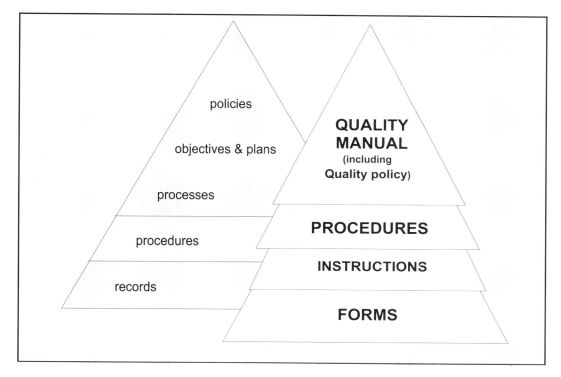

Figure 5.3   Hierarchy of documentation

Throughout the quality manual there should be references to *procedures* which form the second level in the hierachy of documentation. Conceptually a procedure is *'a defined way of progressing a course of action or policy'*. Procedures are the practical way in which policies are translated into action and are often called SOP's or standard operating procedures. The quality policy should refer to management, quality evaluation, health and safety, and laboratory methods etc. and procedures are needed which relate to the same areas.

In the same way that the Quality Manual refers to procedures, so procedures can contain references to *(working) instructions*. This third level of documentation involves the practical day to day work instructions that are needed near the work situation for easy reference. For example they might describe, starting up or closing down a haematology analyzer, a microbiology plate pouring machine, or a recipe for staining a slide. Instructions can be part of a procedure or can be referred to in a procedure and published separately, or be in the document and published separately. The advantage of having them separate is that changes to instructions do not then require a change to the procedure.

The final level in the hierachy of documentation are the *forms*. These are the documents on which records are made that *'provide the evidence that a course of action or policy has been progressed'*. These forms and the records made on them are a crucial part of quality management, they are the evidence that a procedure and/or related instructions have been carried out.

If the procedure or instructions require something to be recorded on a standard form the form must be referred to in the procedure. The forms or records do not necessarily have to be created as 'hard copy' (a paper record). A record (an electronic record) can be created by completing a form on a computer screen placed in the laboratory or consultant's office, by anybody who has the correct authorization identity. Records, whether hard copy or electronic, have to be readily accessible for inspection. In a medical laboratory, request forms and test reports are examples of such documentation and will be discussed further in Chapter 9.

Examples of the use of forms will be given throughout the remainder of the book. Records of any information or data such as patients results, minutes of meetings, quality control data or the result of an audit should be made on forms of an approved format and not on the backs of envelopes or the cuffs of laboratory coats.

A practical example of this hierarchy of documentation, would be a statement in the quality policy requiring *'the use of examination procedures that will ensure the highest achievable quality of all tests performed'* (Figure 4.6). A procedure produced as a result of such a policy statement might be a procedure for measuring HbA1c. In the quality manual, reference would be made to where a list of examination procedures can be found. The procedure might refer to working instructions for starting the HbA1c analyzer and for closing it down and these could be published separately and displayed near the analyzer for easy reference. If the analyzer was interfaced to a laboratory computer then an example of a form would be a computer-generated work sheet to assist with checking-in samples. Additionally, the computer file which holds the patient details and results should be regarded as a record. Such computer-held data needs to be as easily accessible on demand as any paper record.

The term 'protocol' is sometimes used interchangeably with the word 'procedure', particularly when referring to clinical matters. For consistency of approach, the term clinical procedure, rather than clinical protocol, will be used in this book.

All the documents referred to in the hierarchy above must be subject to control as described later in this chapter. In ISO 17025:1999 there is an explanatory note which extends the concept of documents requiring control to include as appropriate: 'specifications, calibration tables, charts, text books, posters, notices, memoranda, software, drawings etc'. It further states that they may be on various media, whether hard copy or electronic, and they may be digital, analog, photographic or written.

At first glance the preparation of required documentation might appear to be a daunting task for a medical laboratory, but in subsequent chapters examples will be given to illustrate that far from being a daunting task, approached in a practical manner it can prove a very effective way of managing the laboratory.

QUALITY MANUAL
'Ideal Standard' clause 4.2.2 Quality manual
In Chapter 4 the purpose, structure and content of a quality manual was discussed. In this chapter the relationship of the quality manual to the organization of procedures is discussed and Figure 5.4 shows the page of the St Elsewhere's quality manual describing the quality management system.

4   QUALITY MANAGEMENT SYSTEM

4.1 GENERAL REQUIREMENT

The Pathology Laboratory has established a quality management system that is described in this Quality Manual and continues to improve its effectiveness by the conduct of an annual management review (see 5.3.7) and by evaluation and quality improvement activities described in section 8 of this manual. Throughout this quality manual the processes required to ensure the effective working of the laboratory are identified and their sequence and interactions defined.

4.2 DOCUMENTATION REQUIREMENTS

4.2.1   General

Pathology laboratory documentation, includes a Quality Manual together with documented statements of policy (5.3.3) [MF-GEN-QualPol], and objectives and plans (5.3.4). The laboratory documents and controls (4.2.3), all procedures and instructions required to ensure effective planning and control of its examination processes (section 7). It maintains and controls process and quality records (4.2.4) and clinical material (4.2.5) with appropriate procedures.

4.2.2   Quality Manual

The Pathology Laboratory maintains a Quality Manual [QM-GEN-QualMan] which is reviewed on an annual basis by the Quality Manager on behalf of the Pathology Management Board and issued under the authority of the Director of Pathology.

4.2.3   Control of documents

The preparation and control of documents is conducted according to the procedure [MP-GEN-DocCtrl].

4.2.4   Control of quality records

The control of process and quality records is conducted according to the procedure [MP-GEN-RecCtrl].

4.2.5   Control of clinical material

The control of clinical material is conducted according to the procedure [MP-GEN-ClnCtrl].

Figure 5.4 Quality manual – the quality management system

ORGANIZATION OF PROCEDURES

The majority of standards used by accreditation bodies require a quality manual to be created. If the standards do not formally require a quality manual it is a good idea to develop one as it serves to introduce the policies and scope of the laboratory facility and to create an organizational structure for documentation. A quality manual can include all the procedures, but in most laboratories this would become an impossibly unwieldy document. Alternatively, the procedures can be referred to in the text and exist as stand alone documents.

In the laboratory of St Elsewhere's Hospital, four distinct types of procedures (and associated instructions and forms), are recognised and these are illustrated in Figure 5.5 in the context of a process-based quality management system for a medical laboratory. Although distinguishing procedures in this way is arbitrary it does provide a logical approach to their management. *Management procedures* are associated with main clauses, 4, 5 and 6 of the 'Ideal Standard'; *Laboratory and Clinical procedures* with main clause 7 and *Quality procedures* with main clause 8.

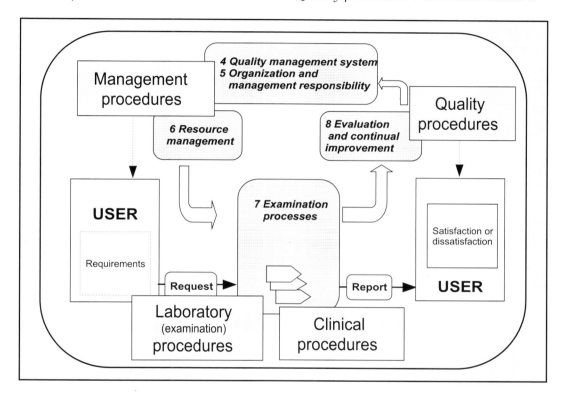

Figure 5.5 Organization of procedures

In practice the procedures are not kept as free standing documents but are often grouped together in books or manuals (hard backed folders). It is possible for each book to have an index and be regarded as volumes of the quality manual. In some disciplines, the laboratory procedures book might be very bulky and would need to be issued in parts to sections of the department. The content of procedures is discussed in later chapters; management procedures in Chapters 4-8, laboratory and clinical procedures in Chapters 9-10, and quality assurance procedures in Chapter 11.

CONTROL OF DOCUMENTS
'Ideal Standard' clause 4.2.3 Control of documents

GENERAL
The major requirements of document control are defined in ISO 9001:2000 and any procedure for document control [MP-GEN-DocCtrl] must set out to fulfil the requirements summarised in Figure 5.6.

Control of documents requires that...

- they are authorized (approved) for adequacy prior to issue

- they are reviewed and updated as required and re-authorized (re-approved)

- any changes and the current revision status are identified

- relevant versions of documents are available at point of use

- they remain legible and identifiable

- documents of external origin are identified and distribution controlled

- unintended use of obsolete documents is prevented

based on ISO 9001:2000 Quality management systems - Requirements

---

Figure 5.6 Requirements for document control

The purpose of the procedure is to establish mechanisms that ensure that all activities or processes in the laboratory use current procedures, instructions and forms, and that an audit of past activities can establish which procedures, instructions and forms were in use at a particular time. Figure 5.7 indicates the contents of the procedure for preparation and control of documentation in the laboratory of St Elsewhere's Hospital.

The preparation and control of a document, whether it is a quality manual, procedure, working instruction or a form should follow a defined process which is shown diagrammatically in Figure 5.8. Such a diagram can usefully be incorporated into a procedure for the preparation and control of documentation.

0	**INTRODUCTION**	**3**	**DOCUMENT CONTROL**
	0.1 Purpose and scope		3.1 Responsibility
	0.2 Responsibility		3.2 Document register
	0.3 References		3.3 Authorization
	0.4 Definitions		3.4 Issue and distribution
	0.5 Documentation		3.5 Removal of redundant documents
1	**DOCUMENT REQUIREMENTS**	**4**	**DOCUMENT CHANGES**
	1.1 The Quality Manual		4.1 Review
	1.2 Procedures		4.2 Revision
	1.3 Instructions		
	1.4 Forms	**5**	**COMPUTER STORAGE**
	1.5 Miscellaneous		
		6	**PRODUCT LIABILITY**
2	**DOCUMENT PREPARATION**		6.1 Manufacturer's method sheets
	2.1 Responsibility		6.2 Change to manufacturer's method
	2.2 Editing and verification		
	2.3 Identification	**7**	**DOCUMENTATION AUDIT**
	2.4 Format		
	2.5 Content		

Figure 5.7 Contents of a procedure for preparation and control of documents [MP-GEN-DocCtrl]

PREPARATION (STEP 1)

GENERAL

Preparation involves three distinct stages, preparation or drafting, editing and validation. If the document is a procedure, instruction or form it is best prepared or designed by the person who regularly carries out the procedure or is familiar with the particular activity e.g. scrutiny of results from external quality assessment schemes. Throughout this section it will be assumed that Microsoft Office or an equivalent is being used, but if documents are created manually then the processes described still need to be followed.

The first action in the preparation of a new document is its registration as a *draft* document. Later in this chapter the distinction between draft, active, inactive and obsolete documents is discussed, as is the nature of the document register and what is registered. A 'dummy' draft document can be registered (Figure 5.8) before it is written, by creating a file with an appropriate filename which, as we shall see later, will be the unique identifier of the document.

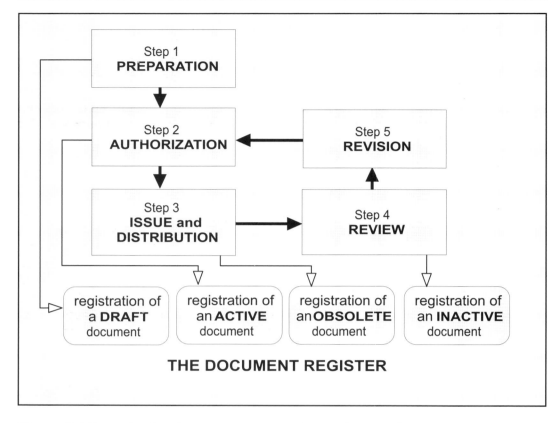

Figure 5.8 Steps in the document preparation and control process

Editing should be a designated task within the laboratory or the department concerned. It involves ensuring that the style of individual documents is similar, throughout a department, or ideally throughout a laboratory. The document should then be subject to validation, preferably by a person who actually uses the procedure.

IDENTIFICATION

It is a requirement of most accreditation standards that documents be uniquely identified. Part of this unique identification is what is called in ISO 15189:2002 'database identification'. This can conveniently be the filename of the document if it is produced by a word processor. Most word processing packages now allow virtually unlimited length filenames but document control packages may place a restriction on the length. For example, Q-pulse, a package produced by Gael Quality restricts the unique identifier to 16 digits. Even with this limitation it is possible to create *'informative filenames'*, that is to say, filenames that provide information as they are read.

In many laboratories, procedures are given alphanumeric filenames such as SOP0038 and this approach requires a secondary index before you can discover what the procedure is about. The informative filename system is used in the laboratory of St Elsewhere's Hospital and Figure 5.9 gives a summary of all the codes in the informative filenames. This table is part of the procedure for preparation and control of documentation. The laboratory has recently introduced the concept of a public document [PD-] to include for example, the Users Handbook [PD-GEN-UserHbk].

At present St Elsewhere's has not combined its document control with St Augustine's and St Bernard's Hospitals, but when it does, this system allows the incorporation of the hospital identifier. St Elsewhere's is limiting its abbreviated titles to 7 digits in anticipation of a merger. If the hospital identifier is never used then the abbreviated title can be 9 digits long. Whether it is best to have the hospital/location code before the department code or vice versa will depend on how the new organization is structured. If the organization is still hospital based, then the order shown in Figure 5.9 is appropriate, but if it is department based i.e, the Department of Biochemistry is organized across all hospitals, the department code should come before the hospital/location code.

Type of document	Hospital/location	Department	Abbreviated title of procedure
XX-	**X-**	**XXX-**	Letters or numbers maximum 7 digits

QM = Quality manual
MP = Management procedure
MI = Management instruction
MF = Management form
 	
LP = Laboratory procedure
LI = Laboratory instruction
      (working instruction)
LF = Laboratory form
 	
CP = Clinical procedure
CF = Clinical form
 	
QP = Quality procedure
QF = Quality form
 	
PD = Public document
	E = St Elsewhere's
	      Hospital
	A = St Augustine's
	      Hospital
	B = St Bernard's
	      Hospital
	1 = EAB
	2 = EA
	3 = EB
	4 = AB
		GEN = General
		BIO = Biochemistry
		HAE = Haematology
		BTR = Blood Transfusion
		MIC = Microbiology
		HIS = Histopathology
		MOR = Mortuary
		OFF = Office
			For example :
			
			DocCtrl =
			Document control
			& preparation
			
			PersMan =
			Personnel
			management

Figure 5.9 Document identification – informative filenames

The International Standards, ISO 17025:1999 and ISO 15189:2002 require other items to form the unique identification of a document. These are listed in Figure

5.10, together with an indication of which items are expected to be present on each page of a draft or active document.

St Elsewhere's Hospital Trust	Edition: 1.0	Filename: MP-GEN-PathMan
	Author: J. Qualiman	Authorized by: W.Jaggard
PATHOLOGY LABORATORY	Date of issue: 05/01/2001	Page: 2/12

Item of unique identification	Draft document	Active document
Title	+	+
Database identification (informative filename)	+	+
Page/total number of pages	+	+
Edition number	+	+
Date of issue or revision date	-	+
Authority for issue	-	+
Author	+	+

Figure 5.10 Document identification required on each page

FORMAT
There are a number of features in word processing packages that enable documents to be well designed and have features added to their text automatically and under control of the document creation process. The *header* and *footer* facility allows information to be put at the top and bottom of every page in a document.

At St Elsewhere's, with the exception of the title, the unique identification information is put in the header, as shown for the pathology management procedure [MP-GEN-PathMan] (top of Figure 5.10). It would be possible to include the title in the header as well as on a title page, but by using 'informative filenames' the information is already present in a readable form. These items of unique identification can be placed into the header automatically using the *Insert/Autotext* and *Insert/Field* facilities in Microsoft Word. The significance of each item is discussed later in this chapter. The left hand side of the header in Figure 5.10 also gives the name of the host organization and department or laboratory. If the organization or department has a logo this can be incorporated into the header if desired.

Most forms and instructions will be single pages with a fixed format and do not require a front (title) page. However, procedures do require a front page; it should have a clear succinct title together with a table giving the location of copies and document review history. These latter items can be dispensed with if an electronic document control system is used. In this situation it may be possible to accommodate the contents (see below), on the front page. A front page is illustrated for the Quality Manual in Chapter 4, Figure 4.11. It is useful if the title can be brief, for example, 'A Procedure for the Measurement of Urine Potassium', can be shortened to 'Urine potassium' or even 'UrineK' allowing an informative file name, [LP-BIO-UrineK].

CONTENT

The preceding paragraphs dealt with the information which should appear on each page of any document and the front page of a procedure. The second page for a procedure is usually the *table of contents*, e.g. Figure 4.2. The content of the body of a document will vary in accordance with the type of document. It is helpful if the opening pages of a procedure have a standard structure. Figure 5.11 shows the structure for the introductory section of the procedure for document preparation and control [MP-GEN-DocCtrl] which has five sub-sections.

Purpose and scope, describes the purpose of the procedure and the area of laboratory activity to which it applies. In the case of the example in Figure 5.11 the procedure applies to the whole laboratory, whereas a quality procedure for the management of external quality assessment schemes in the Department of Histopathology [QP-HIST-EQAMan] would have the same scope as a similar procedure for Haematology, but would only refer to Histopathology.

Responsibility defines who is responsible for implementation of the procedure and to whom they report. *References* should include a reference to the appropriate clause of the accreditation standard and any source material that has guided the preparation of the procedure. The *Definitions* section is used to define any words that have a specific technical meaning in the context of the procedure. Finally, *Documentation* refers to any forms used in the implementation of the procedure. It is these completed forms (records) that provide evidence of the conduct of the procedure. This section can also include references to instructions or other procedures to be used in conjunction with the procedure.

The content of the rest of the procedure will be determined by the nature of the procedure. In the case of the procedure for document preparation and control, the whole content is shown in Figure 5.7. The most difficult part of writing a procedure is determining the structure of the content and throughout the rest of the book, examples of content will be provided. A good way of monitoring the structure of a procedure in terms of headings and sub-headings is by using the auto-contents function in Microsoft Word *(Insert/Contents/Table of Contents)*. It is advisable to create sub-headings only to the second decimal place (e.g. 3.2.2) or preferably to one decimal place (e.g. 3.2) and thereafter use a), b), c) etc.

St Elsewhere's Hospital Trust	Edition: 1.0	Filename: MP-GEN-DocCtrl
	Author: J. Qualiman	Authorized by: W.Jaggard
PATHOLOGY LABORATORY	Date of issue: 05/02/2001	Page: 3/12

0   INTRODUCTION

0.1   Purpose and scope

To define the procedure for preparation and control of all documents, including the Quality Manual [QM-GEN-QualMan], procedures, instructions and forms and other miscellaneous documents, such as manufacturer's manuals. This procedure is operable throughout the Pathology Laboratory.

0.2   Responsibility

The Quality Manager liases with the Director of Pathology for the implementation and maintenance of this procedure and reports directly to the Director of Diagnostic and Therapeutic Medicine.

The Quality Manager works closely with members of the Quality and Accreditation Committee and other appropriate members of staff in implementing and maintaining this procedure.

0.3   References

'Ideal Standard' clause 4.2.3 Control of documents

ISO 9001:2000 4.2.3 Control of documents

ISO 17025:1999 4.3 Document control

ISO 15189:2002 4.3 Document control

CPA(UK)Ltd A8 Document control

0.4   Definitions

Quality manager: person in charge of co-ordinating the management of quality and compliance with accreditation standards

Responsible manager: person responsible for overseeing the preparation and control of documentation in particular areas of the Pathology Laboratory

Author: the person responsible for the preparation of any document

Authorizer: the person responsible for authorization of a document

Authorization: the process of final checking of a document, prior to issue

0.5   Documentation

[MP-GEN-QPulse4]   Q-Pulse, Version 4, Users manual

[MF-GEN-DocAmnd] Document amendment form

[MF-GEN-DocNotf]   Document notification form

Figure 5.11 Procedure content – 0 Introduction

AUTHORIZATION (STEP 2)

The second step is authorization (sometimes called approval), of the document. It is at this point that the document moves from a draft to being an active document (a document ready to be put into use) and has to be registered in the document register as an active document (Figure 5.8, Step 2). The responsibility for authorization is normally that of the person in a direct line management relationship. For example, at St Elsewhere's the author of the Quality Manual is John Qualiman, and the authorization is done by the Director of Pathology, Dr W Jaggard. It is at this stage that the name of the person authorizing the document can be entered into the header of the document. If it was a technical procedure prepared by a member of staff from a section of Biochemistry, the authorizer should be the section head. It is important that the preparation of procedures and authorization goes as far down the management structure as possible, in order that the procedure reflects real knowledge of the process involved. Although authorization is described as a separate step it is normally immediately followed by issue and distribution.

ISSUE AND DISTRIBUTION (STEP 3)

Whether the issue and distribution is done manually, or using an electronic document preparation and control system, it is at this stage that the date of issue should be added. An alternative is to issue it with the date of revision. At St Elsewhere's where all documents are reviewed annually, all documents are given an issue date Inspection of the issue date and the document review history panel on the front page will quickly establish whether the document has been reviewed at an appropriate date. All copies that are issued as active documents (whether in electronic or hard copy) should have all the data shown in the right hand column of Figure 5.10 completed. The word 'edition' is used throughout this text rather than issue or version, as meaning 'one of a number of printings issued at separate times with alterations and amendments incorporated'. Some standards require the actual signatures of the author and authorizer, but this should not be necessary in a medical laboratory using a suitable electronic document control system.

Whilst the document is in draft form any copies in circulation should be printed on **plain white paper** and are considered to be UNCONTROLLED documents. All active documents can be printed on **paper of a distinctive colour** and this paper should only be available for that purpose. It is useful to choose a color that photocopies poorly to avoid illicit copies being made. These documents are CONTROLLED documents. It is a good rule to issue the minimum number of paper copies required. If further paper copies are made of authorized and issued documents over and above those on the official circulation list, these must be printed on plain white paper and stamped UNCONTROLLED COPY.

REVIEW (STEP 4)

At first sight the prospect of reviewing a very large number of documents can be very daunting until it becomes clear that review does not imply revision. The purpose of reviewing a document is to ascertain its continuing 'fitness for purpose'. If it is still fit for its intended purpose then a record needs to be made of the date of review and the reviewer on the front page, document review panel (see Figure 4.11) of issued hard copies and in the document register. In rare cases, for example if an examination, and therefore its procedure, is temporarily withdrawn from use then the active document can become an inactive document (Figure 5.8).

REVISION (STEP 5)

Whilst a document is in use certain imperfections will come to light. In the case of instructions and forms, the document can very easily be revised and a new edition issued. The old edition then becomes an *obsolete* document (Figure 5.8). If instructions and forms are simply referred to in procedures rather than incorporated into the procedure, they can be revised independently of the procedure and vice versa.

However, for a procedure in use, minor changes are a more complex problem. The problem has three dimensions, the first, is how to control the changes, the second is how to make the changes and the third is how to indicate the changes to the user. If the document control system is entirely electronic, as is the case with Q-Pulse, then in theory it is possible to work in a paperless environment and issue no paper copies of any procedure. In practice, however, most staff like to have ready access to a paper copy, and keeping the active paper and electronic copies identical implies issuing new hard copies whenever changes are made. In Q-Pulse it is possible to keep a file of proposed minor changes to a procedure that can then be consulted when it is reviewed and a decision made as to whether the changes are important enough to merit the revision and issuing of a new edition.

At St Elsewhere's these minor changes or amendments are recorded on a document amendment form [MF-GEN-DocAmnd] kept at the back of every procedure issued as hard copy (Figure 5.12). The changes made have to follow strict rules: (a) the amendment must be authorized by a section head and must be considered minor, (b) the amendment must be underlined and an asterisk placed in the margin alongside the amendment, (c) ten or less amendments can be made before the procedure is revised, and (d) any major amendment must lead to an immediate full revision of the procedure and its re-issue as a subsequent edition.

A minor amendment is an amendment that does not materially affect the operation of the procedure, such as correction of a spelling mistake or incorrect bolding. The figure for the number of amendments which can be made before revision is arbitrary, but is intended to prevent the document becoming too untidy. Documents in use must maintain their quality, particularly with regard to legibility

DOCUMENT AMENDMENT FORM

RECORD FILENAME	

Number	Date	Page no.	Amendment	Authorized by:
1				
2				
3				
4				
5				
6				
7				
8				
9				
10				

- The amendment must be authorized by the section head
- The amendment must be underlined and an asterisk written in the margin alongside the change *(liquid paper must not be used)*
- Ten or less minor amendments can be made before the procedure is revised
- Major changes must result in the immediate review of the procedure

Figure 5.12 Content of a document amendment form [MF-GEN-DocAmnd]

CONTROL OF DOCUMENTS FROM AN EXTERNAL SOURCE

Documents which originate from external sources such as equipment manuals, may also need to be registered as controlled documents. For example, the procedure for document control and preparation (MP-GEN-DocCtrl) in the laboratory at St Elsewhere's makes reference throughout to the Q-Pulse, Version 4, Users Manual, and copies of this manual are made into controlled documents by registering them in Q-Pulse and giving them a procedure name (MP-GEN-QPulse4). Each copy would then have a label stuck on it with a minimum of identification data (Figure 5.13). Only copies of the manual that have such a label attached are regarded as active documents. If it was the manual for an HbA1c Analyzer called a B200, it could be registered as [LP-BIO-B200Man].

Filename:	MP-GEN-QPulse4
Authorized by:	J Qualiman
Date of issue:	05/01/2001
Copy:	2/5
Title:	Q-Pulse Version 4 Users Manual

Figure 5.13 Label for a controlled document from an external source

THE DOCUMENT REGISTER

The first decision with regard to the document register or master index of documentation is to decide whether the document register should be a manual paper record, a homemade spreadsheet or database, or an off the shelf (albeit customisable) commercial product. This is perhaps the most important decision that any laboratory can make in preparing for accreditation. The author has experience of all three approaches but would unequivocally opt for the off the shelf commercial product providing it was well tested and a reasonable price. Q-Pulse, produced by Gael Quality, is increasingly being used in the UK and Ireland. It is robust, reasonably priced, user friendly and is being progressively developed. It can be downloaded and used on a 30 day trial basis from the Gael Quality website (www.gaelquality.com).

At St Elsewhere's Hospital the laboratory uses the features of the Document (Control) Module of Q-Pulse not only to register the identification data shown in Figure 5.10 but also (a) to control access to the document, to determine the author and authorizer (b) to link it to other relevant documents (c) to link it to particular processes, standards, departments etc to enable audit. This concept is illustrated in Figure 5.14 with reference to the procedure for document control [MP-GEN-DocCtrl].

Unique identification (Q-pulse terms)	Data entered
Title (Title)	Preparation and control of documents
Data based identification (Number)	MP-GEN-DocCtrl
Edition number (Revision)	1.0
Date of issue (Active date)	05/02/2001
Authority for issue (Approval level)	W Jaggard
Author (Update responsibility)	J Qualiman
Other control data	**Data entered**
Status (Status)	Active
Review date (Review date)	05/02/2002
Change details (Change details)	Edition 1.0 prepared for accreditation
Change number (Change number)	MP01 [links to document recording required changes based on MF-GEN-DocAmnd]
Document distribution (Document distribution)	[links to names of authorized users]
Document properties	**Data entered**
Area of Standards (Areas of Standard)	'Ideal Standard' 4.2.3 Control of documents
	ISO 9001:2000 4.2.3 Control of documents
	ISO 17025:1999 4.3 Document control
	ISO 15189:2002 4.3 Document control
	CPA(UK)Ltd A8 Document control
Departments (Departments)	Pathology Laboratory
Documentation (References)	MP-GEN-Qpulse4
	MF-GEN-DocAmnd
	MF-GEN-DocNotf
Area of process (area of process)	Document control

Figure 5.14 Functions of a document register

CONTROL OF RECORDS
'Ideal Standard' clause 4.2.4 Control of records

GENERAL
In ISO 9001:2000 it says 'records shall be established and maintained to provide evidence of conformity to requirements and of the effective running of the QMS'. It further stipulates that they shall remain legible, readily identifiable and retrievable and that a procedure be established to define the controls necessary for identification, storage, protection, retrieval, retention time and disposition of records. At St Elsewhere's the procedure for control of records [MP-GEN-RecCtrl] aims to fulfil these stipulations and its contents are shown in Figure 5.15.

0	**INTRODUCTION**	3	**IDENTIFICATION AND INDEXING**

0 **INTRODUCTION**
- 0.1 Purpose and scope
- 0.2 Responsibility
- 0.3 References
- 0.4 Definitions
- 0.5 Documentation

1 **GENERAL**
- 1.1 Requirements of the laboratory
- 1.2 Requirements of St Elsewhere's Hospital Trust
- 1.3 Requirements of legislation

2 **RECORD TYPE AND RETENTION TIMES**
- 2.1 Organization and management
- 2.2 Resource management
- 2.3 Pre-examination, examination and post-examination processes
- 2.4 Evaluation and quality improvement

3 **IDENTIFICATION AND INDEXING**
- 3.1 Identification
- 3.2 Indexing

4 **CONFIDENTIALITY AND SECURITY**
- 4.1 Confidentiality
- 4.2 Security of hard copy
- 4.3 Security of electronic media

5 **STORAGE AND RETRIEVAL**
- 5.1 On-site
- 5.2 Off-site
- 5.3 External contractors

6 **RELEASE AND DISPOSAL**
- 6.1 Release to patients
- 6.2 Release to third parties
- 6.3 On-site
- 6.4 External contractors

7 **AUDIT OF RECORD CONTROL**

Figure 5.15 Contents of a procedure for control of records [MP-GEN-RecCtrl]

ISO 9001:2000, being a quality standard, simply refers to retention and storage of quality records, whereas the laboratory focused standards ISO 17025:1999 and ISO 15189:2002 refer to the retention and control of quality and process records and in the case of ISO 15189:2002 clinical material as well (see Chapter 9).

Whether the requirement is for control of clinical material or records, there are three distinct issues to be considered, firstly, are the records being retained going to serve a useful purpose, for example to reconstruct an examination, or to audit corrective action. Secondly, what are the relevant retention times, and thirdly how should the material be kept.

RETENTION TIMES
In order to decide appropriate retention times a number of factors require consideration (Figure 5.16). The primary concern should be the ability to reconstruct, in as far as it is possible, the sequence of events from the receipt of a request and specimen to the issuing of the result of the examination as a report. This activity is termed vertical audit and is discussed in Chapter 11.

- Review and confirmation of examination processes after the report has been received by the requesting clinician

- Time interval between assessment visits by the accreditation body

- National legislation and regulation

- Retention for research purposes

Figure 5.16 Factors affecting the retention times of clinical material and records

There will be special circumstances where retention times will be at variance with a laboratory's normal practice, for example, if the laboratory is undertaking examinations as part of a clinical trial then particular requirements may be set by the organization undertaking the trial. The impact of legislation will vary in different countries and if, for example, a manufacturer's method is altered by a laboratory, the liability under consumer protection legislation will shift from the manufacturer to the laboratory and detailed records of validation studies will need to be kept in case of litigation. Liabilty to prosecution has to be a major factor in determining retention times.

Figures 5.17 and 5.18 provide information on recommended minimum retention times compiled from a report from the Royal College of Pathologists (RCPath) entitled 'The Retention and Storage of Pathological Records and Archives' and the NPAAC guidelines 'Retention of Laboratory Records and Diagnostic Material', and compares it with practice in St Elsewhere's. In the figure a single asterisk (NPAAC) and double asterisk (St Elsewhere's) indicate the influence of the time interval between assessments by accreditation bodies, in that the accreditation bodies might wish to examine any process that has taken place since the last visit. The records being kept are categorised against the main clauses of the 'Ideal Standard'.

In addition to retaining the records shown in Figures 5.17 and 5.18, copies of inactive and obsolete procedures, instructions, forms and public documents should be retained.

Section of 'Ideal Standard'	NPACC (Australia)	RCPath (UK)	St Elsewhere's Hospital Trust
5 ORGANIZATION & MANAGEMENT RESPONSIBILITY			
Minutes of meetings	-	-	4 years**
Objectives and plans	-	-	4 years**
Management reviews	-	-	Permanently
6 RESOURCE MANAGEMENT			
6.2 Personnel			
Personnel records	Employment plus 3 years*	-	Employment plus 4 years**
6.3 Premises			
Fire/ Health & Safety/ Radiological Protection Certificates	3 years*	10 years or until superseded	4 years**
6.4 Equipment, information systems and reagents			
Equipment maintenance and service records	Life of the machine plus 3 years*	Length of life (minimum 10 years)	Equipment life plus 4 years**
8 EVALUATION and QUALITY IMPROVEMENT			
Internal audit reports, including Health & Safety	-	-	4 years**
EQA scheme reports	3 years*	2 years	4 years**
External agency reports	-	10 years or until superseded	4 years**
Quality improvement records	-	-	4 years**

Figure 5.17 Retention of management and quality records

IDENTIFICATION AND INDEXING

When a form is completed it becomes a record. The informative filename of the form and the control details in the header of the form remain unchanged (Figure 6.7 illustrates this for a job description). If the record created is a paper record then it is generally filed in a specific place, in for example, date or alphabetical order. Such a record might be a maintenance schedule for a piece of equipment. However, if the record is created and stored electronically then it is useful to store it under a *record filename* which will be recorded in the body of the form as distinct from the header of the form (see Figure 6.7).

Section of 'Ideal Standard'	NPACC (Australia)	RCPath (UK)	St Elsewheres' Hospital Trust
7 EXAMINATION PROCESSES			
7.1 Pre-examination process			
Request forms	7 years In cases of children, retain until the child reaches age 25	1 month	3 months (plus scanned record permanently)
Patient correspondence	As above	As above	As above
7.2 Examination process			
Laboratory procedures (LP-) & Instructions (LI-)	While methods current + 3 years*	Permanently	While methods current + 4 years**
Request forms with results	See request forms	2 years	4 years**
Day books	See request forms-	2 years	Not applicable
Work sheets	See request forms	Same length of time as related specimens or preparations	4 years**
Internal quality control records	3 years*	Permanently	4 years**
Method validation records	-	-	While methods current + 4 years**
Post mortem records	20 years	Permanently	Permanently
Blood Bank records	20 years	11 years	20 years
7.3 Post-examination process			
Reports	Permanent	6 months for operational purposes	Permanently

Figure 5.18 Retention of examination records

Although it is necessary in some electronic document management systems such as Q-Pulse to limit the length of the informative filename to 16 digits this same constraint does not apply to the filename of the record made using a form. At St Elsewhere's a procedure is followed in which the record filename consists of the informative filename of the form, followed by a hash symbol # and the information used to uniquely identify the record.

Figure 5.19 shows examples of this approach. It is desirable that the forms used in certain key areas, such as minutes and job descriptions are the same throughout pathology and have the same informative filenames, e.g. for job descriptions [MF-GEN-JobDesc]. However, if records created using the forms are created by a particular departmental activity then the MF-GEN- in the filename can be changed to, for example, MF-HAE-.

RELEASE AND DISPOSAL

Sections 6.1 and 6.2 of the procedure for control of records [MP-GEN-RecCtrl] (Figure 5.15) concern the release of records to patients and to third parties. In the United Kingdom, the Information Commissioner has produced guidance on the Data Protection Act 1998 entitled 'Use and Disclosure of Health Data' that provides the current parameters for action at St Elsewhere's. It is important to appreciate that the Act 'applies fully to all patient records whether they are held on computer or in paper files, and whether they consist of hand written notes or X-rays'. Similar advice will be found in different jurisdictions. Otherwise destructive disposal must be secure and in accordance with the waste disposal procedures in the owning institution.

FORMS INTO RECORDS

Throughout the rest of the book further examples will be given of how records are created using controlled forms and how this is the evidence that makes internal audit possible. An example of how this can be used within an organization, to further the orderly conduct of business, is the keeping of minutes. At St Elsewhere's, minutes of all meetings are kept using a form [MF-GEN-Minutes], a partially completed example of which is shown in Figure 5.20. Three issues are of great importance for the successful recording of meetings. Firstly, the numbering of each minute and the minute number/year system (e.g. 23/2002) is very effective and better in the author's view than the minute number/meeting number (e.g. 23/1) system.

Secondly, minutes should record decisions and not every individual contribution to the discussion. It can be seen from Figure 5.20 that there is no space for an 'Acceptance of the minutes of the last meeting', this is because at St Elsewhere's the chairman or secretary of the meeting write the minutes at the time and they are agreed at the time of the meeting as a correct record. This is not too difficult if only decisions are recorded and saves the hours of wasted time, that all readers of this book will have endured, having the accuracy of the minutes of the last meeting often endlessly contested, particularly by people who were not there!! Finally, where the recorded minute requires some action the person responsible for taking action and a timescale should be recorded.

FORM		Corresponding RECORD	
Informative filename	**Name of form**	**Record filename**	**Record**
MF-GEN-Minutes	Minutes	MF-GEN-Minutes # Brd 02Mar'02	Minutes of the Pathology Board held on the 2nd March 2002
		MF-GEN-Minutes #H&S 04May'02	Minutes of the Health and Safety Committee held on the 4th May 2002
		MF-HAE-Minutes #Dept 03Jan'01	Minutes of the Haematology Department held on the 3rd January 2001
MF-GEN-DocAmnd	Document amendment form	MF-GEN-DocAmnd #MP-GEN- PersMan	Document amendment form attached to the procedure for personnel management
MF-GEN-JobDesc	Job descriptions	MF-GEN-JobDesc # CompMan	Job description for a Pathology Computer Manager
		MF-HIS-JobDesc # ConHisto	Job description for a Consultant Histopathologist
MF-GEN-JntRev	Annual joint review form	MF-BIO-JntRev # JohnStartup 04-Jan'02	Annual joint review record for John Startup, 4th January 2002
MF-GEN-TrnRec	Training record	MF-BIO-TrnRec # JohnStartup 03-Jan'01	Training record for John Startup, 3th January 2001

Figure 5.19 Forms into records

MINUTES	
RECORD FILENAME	MF-GEN-Minutes#PathBrd 02-03-02

Title of Meeting	Pathology board	**Date of meeting**	2nd March 2002

Present

(**THIS IS GUIDANCE**, Enter names)

Apologies for absence

(**THIS IS GUIDANCE**, Enter names)

Items continuing from the previous minutes

(**THIS IS GUIDANCE,** each minute should be numbered sequentially throughout the year and have a title in bold type)	(**THIS IS GUIDANCE**, Action required should be recorded and a time for execution included)
001/2001 Car parking	
The Laboratory manager will investigate the allocation of car parking space	Report for next meeting on 4th April 2002

New Minutes

009/2002 Storage space	
An investigation of all storage space used by the laboratory should be carried out and a brief report prepared by the Health and Safety committee	Report for meeting on 5th May 2002
010/2002	
The Chairman of the Trust Board will visit the laboratory at 12.00 on the 6th June 2002 to open the new patient reception area, to be followed by a buffet lunch for all staff. All available members of the Pathology Board to be present	Presence on 6th June 2002

Date of the next meeting(s)

(**THIS IS GUIDANCE**, try to arrange dates of meetings for a year or at minimum the next two meetings)

Figure 5.20 Partially completed minutes for St Elsewhere's Pathology Management Board [MF-GEN-Minutes#PathBrd 2Mar'02}

CONTROL OF CLINICAL MATERIAL
'Ideal Standard' clause 4.2.5 Control of clinical material
This topic will be discussed in Chapter 9, Examination process.

Chapter 6

Personnel

INTRODUCTION
'Ideal Standard' clause 6.2 Personnel
The way in which an organization attracts, develops, motivates and retains staff determines the quality of the service it provides and whether it is responsive to the changing needs of its users. There are marked differences between the different International Standards with regard to personnel requirements. In ISO 9001:2000, clause 6.2, *'Human resources'*, requires personnel to be competent in terms of appropriate education, training, skills and experience and looks to competence and awareness being established and training given. ISO 17025:1999 embraces these requirements but emphasises the need for adequate supervision of staff undergoing training, for job descriptions, contracts, and personnel/staff records. It specifies the need for appropriate qualifications, training, experience and/or demonstrated skills for specific tasks.

In ISO 9001:2000 and ISO 17025:1999 respectively, no attempt is made to be prescriptive about top management or laboratory management, in terms of specified arrangements or particular qualifications. ISO 15189:2002 as an International Standard specifically for medical laboratories is more prescriptive, defining laboratory management as 'those persons who manage the activities of the laboratory headed by the laboratory director'. The laboratory director is then defined as 'a person or persons who have the competence to assume the responsibility and authority for the laboratory', and various specific responsibilities are assigned to this person or persons, albeit with the power of delegation. These competencies are discussed later in the chapter.

This chapter looks at three distinct aspects of personnel management. Firstly, staff structures and accountability, staff numbers and job evaluation, recruitment, selection, and induction, job descriptions and personnel records. Secondly, competence, awareness and training and the role of an annual joint review and thirdly, communication with staff.

Figure 6.1 illustrates the inter-connectivity of the different aspects of personnel management as detailed in Clause 6.2 of the 'Ideal Standard'.

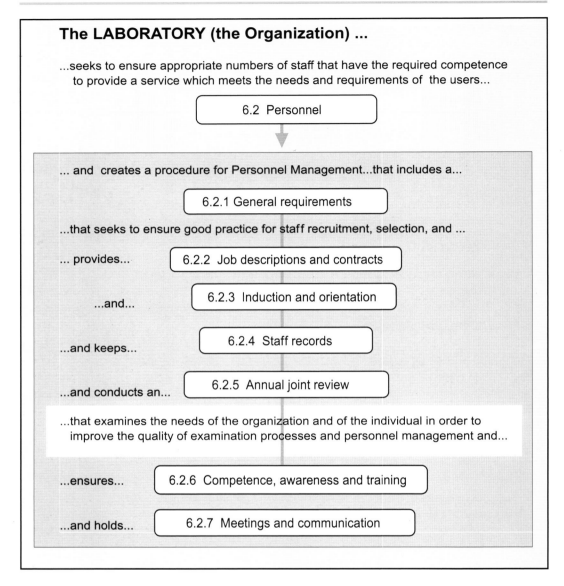

The LABORATORY (the Organization) ...

...seeks to ensure appropriate numbers of staff that have the required competence to provide a service which meets the needs and requirements of the users...

6.2 Personnel

... and creates a procedure for Personnel Management...that includes a...

6.2.1 General requirements

...that seeks to ensure good practice for staff recruitment, selection, and ...

... provides...   6.2.2 Job descriptions and contracts

...and...   6.2.3 Induction and orientation

...and keeps...   6.2.4 Staff records

...and conducts an...   6.2.5 Annual joint review

...that examines the needs of the organization and of the individual in order to improve the quality of examination processes and personnel management and...

...ensures...   6.2.6 Competence, awareness and training

...and holds...   6.2.7 Meetings and communication

Figure 6.1 Clause 6.2 of the 'Ideal Standard' – Personnel management

GENERAL REQUIREMENTS

'Ideal Standard' clause 6.2.1 General requirement

The scope of ISO 9004:2000, 'Quality management systems – Guidelines for performance improvements', describes its role as providing 'guidelines beyond the requirements given in ISO 9001:2000 in order to consider both the effectiveness and efficiency of a QMS and consequently the potential for improvement of an organization'. In clause 6.2 of ISO 9004:2000, some important principles for the involvement of people in the work of an organization are enumerated (Figure 6.2). The laboratory at St Elsewhere's embraces these principles in its Quality Policy (Figure 4.6), where it states that it is committed to 'staff recruitment, training, development and retention at all levels to provide a full and effective service to its users'.

The laboratory should encourage involvement and development of its people by...

- providing ongoing training and career planning

- defining their responsibilities and authorities

- setting individual and departmental objectives, managing process performance and evaluating results

- facilitating involvement in objective setting and decision making

- recognising and rewarding

- open, two way communication of information

- continually review the needs of its people

- creating conditions that encourage innovation

- ensuring effective team work

- communicating suggestions and opinions

- using measurements of people's satisfaction, and investigation of reasons why people join and leave an organization

based on ISO 9004:2000 Quality management systems – Guidelines for performance improvements

---

Figure 6.2 The involvement of people in the work of an organization

Legislation and regulations in different countries will affect certain aspects of personnel management. However, there is an emerging consensus of good practice that is reflected in Figure 6.2 and in the well balanced advice that can be found on the website (www.acas.org.uk) of the Advisory, Conciliation and Arbitration Service (ACAS) in the UK. ACAS is a public body funded by the taxpayer and one of its roles is to encourage people to work together effectively. This principle is expressed in the ACAS standard 'Working Together' and in the 'Employment Handbook, A-Z of Work'. Material detailed in this chapter and in Appendix 2 Further reading, is available, mostly free of charge, from their website.

PROCEDURES FOR PERSONNEL MANAGEMENT

The extent to which the laboratory has its own procedures for personnel management and the extent to which they are determined by the parent body or host organization will vary from laboratory to laboratory. For example some laboratories will undertake their own recruitment and selection and in others it will be a shared activity. The content of the personnel procedure used in the laboratory at St Elsewhere's is shown in Figure 6.3. Items marked with an asterisk are those undertaken jointly with the Human Resources (Personnel) Department of the hospital and where, for brevity, reference is made to hospital procedures, an up to date set of which is kept by the Business Manager.

---

0 INTRODUCTION
    0.1 Purpose and scope
    0.2 Responsibility
    0.3 References
    0.4 Definitions
    0.5 Documentation

1 RECRUITMENT AND RETENTION*
    1.1 Relationship to Human Resources Department
    1.2 Advertisements
    1.3 Interviews
    1.4 Miscellaneous

2 JOB DESCRIPTIONS AND CONTRACTS*
    2.1 Responsibility
    2.2 Terms and conditions of employment
    2.3 Person specifications [MF-GEN-PerSpec]
    2.4 Job descriptions [MF-GEN-JobDesc]

3 INDUCTION AND ORIENTATION*
    3.1 Responsibility
    3.2 Hospital induction programme
    3.3 Laboratory induction programme
    3.4 Induction record [MF-GEN-StafInd]

4 RECORDS*
    4.1 Responsibility
    4.2 Relationship to Human Resources Department
    4.3 Staff record [MF-GEN-StafRec]

5 ANNUAL JOINT REVIEW
    5.1 Responsibility
    5.2 Content and process
    5.3 Joint review record [MF-GEN-JntRev]

6 COMPETENCE, AWARENESS AND TRAINING
    6.1 Responsibility
    6.2 Competence testing and training records [MF-GEN-TrngRec]
    6.3 Training programmes
    6.4 Registration of continuous professional development
    6.5 Study leave

7 MEETINGS AND COMMUNICATIONS
    7.1 Departmental meetings
    7.2 Two way communication

8 DISCIPLINARY AND GRIEVANCE PROCEDURES*

Figure 6.3 Content of a procedure for personnel management [MP-GEN-PersMan]

STAFF STRUCTURE AND ACCOUNTABILITY

In Chapter 4 the need to clearly define the responsibilities, relationships and authorities of staff and the use of organizational charts was discussed. Pages 6 and 7 (Figures 4.15 and 4.16) of the Quality Manual of the laboratory at St Elsewhere's provide charts which show both the structure of the laboratory and the accountability of senior staff to the Director of Pathology. Organization charts that show staff accountability are sometimes termed accountability charts, but in this text the 'organization chart' is used to cover both laboratory structure and staff accountability. Such a chart can be a valuable part of a job description and can be complemented by a written description of staff relationships. An example of such a chart is shown in the job description of a Medical Laboratory Assistant (Figure 6.7), employed in the Department of Haematology at St Elsewhere's.

STAFF RESOURCES AND JOB EVALUATION

It is always a vexed question in any industry as to how many staff are required to do a particular job. ISO 17025:1999, clause 4.1 'Organization', requires that 'the laboratory shall have managerial and technical personnel with the authority and resources needed to carry out their duties…' and ISO 15189:2002, clause 5.1 'Personnel', includes a requirement that, 'there shall be adequate staff resources to undertake the work required…'. CPA(UK)Ltd, Standard B2 Staffing, states, 'laboratory management shall ensure that there are appropriate numbers of staff, with the required education and training, to meet the demands of the service and appropriate national legislation and regulations'. Similarly NPAAC, Draft Standard 2, Staffing, supervision and consultation says, 'there shall be sufficient pathologists, scientific, technical and support staff all of whom shall have documented appropriate qualifications, training and experience to conduct the work of the laboratory'.

This single requirement constitutes the most difficult task that faces an assessor from an accreditation body trying to determine compliance to standards. Whereas it is relatively easy to ascertain, from records of qualifications and training and from assessments of competence, the fitness of the staff to undertake their assigned work, it is much more difficult to determine whether 'adequate staff resources', 'appropriate numbers' or 'sufficient' staff are employed. It should be possible to establish, by a combination of the professional (technical) experience of an assessor and from norms established by professional bodies, whether a laboratory is adequately staffed. However, this must always be supported by objective observation and assessment of the quality of service provided.

The nature and number of staff required by a laboratory has to be constantly kept under review as the nature and quantity of the work changes, as new technologies make their impact, and new working practices and organizational structures develop. When a member of staff leaves an organization it is always a good point at which to evaluate that job and decide whether it is still appropriate in its current form. The Annual Joint Review discussed later in this chapter is an opportunity to review an individual's training and development needs in relation to changes in the needs of the organization.

STAFF RECRUITMENT AND SELECTION

Often the first contact that a potential employee has with an organization will be through responding to an advertisement in a newspaper or professional journal. The laboratory may also have open days for the general public, co-operate with local schools in arranging work experience for senior pupils, or participate in careers conventions. These contacts are important, particularly in attracting locally recruited staff.

Advertisements should have an attractive format and contain a clear indication on how to obtain further information and who to contact to make an appointment for an informal visit. The information sent to a potential applicant should include a job description, a person specification, information about the laboratory and its host organization, and a job application form.

The role, format, and content of the job description is discussed below. Once a job has been defined, the next task is to create a profile of a person who would be suitable for the post. This profile is often called a person specification and there are a number of different ways in which it can be constructed. Figure 6.4 shows the content of a person specification form completed for a personal secretary to the head of the Haematology department of St Elsewhere's Hospital Trust.

As with minutes of meetings (see Chapter 5), although the informative filename of a controlled form is restricted to 16 digits, the length of the filename of a completed form (a record) is not limited in length. If the informative filename for the person specification form is [MF-GEN-PerSpec], it can then be adjusted to create a record filename for the individual record, in this case MF-HAE-PerSpec#DeptSec, or for example in the case of a Principal Biochemist, MF-BIO-PerSpec#PrinBio.

PERSON SPECIFICATION FORM			
RECORD FILENAME	*MF-HAE-PerSpec#DeptSec*		
1 Job title	*Departmental Secretary*	**2 Location**	*Haematology*

	ESSENTIAL	**DESIRABLE**
3 Impact on other people	*Acceptable bearing and speech.*	*Pleasant manner, bearing and speech.*
4 Qualifications and experience	*GCSE English language or equivalent. Ability to audiotype accurately, and to operate office machines. Experience of general office work.*	*GCSE maths or equivalent. RSA III typing. Experience of using simple statistical information. Experience of staff supervision.*
5 Innate abilities	*Quick to grasp a point.*	*Ability to assess priorities and make decisions.*
6 Motivation	*Personal identification with service given by the department. Interest in efficiency of administration.*	
7 Adjustment	*Steady, self-reliant, good at making friendly relationships with colleagues at all levels.*	*Able to cope with stress and pressure from different user departments.*

Figure 6.4 Completed person specification form [MF-HAE-PerSpec#DeptSec]

JOB DESCRIPTIONS AND CONTRACTS
'Ideal Standard' clause 6.2.2 Job descriptions and contracts

TERMS AND CONDITIONS OF EMPLOYMENT
Employment rights in many countries fall into two categories, statutory rights and contractual rights that together make a contract of employment. This contract is a legally enforceable agreement between two people (parties), which may be verbal or in writing. Written contracts reduce the potential for subsequent disputes. In the UK, employees have statutory rights with regard to written terms and conditions of employment, pay, working hours, holidays and time off, maternity/paternity leave, belonging to a trade union, health and safety and not to be

discriminated against. The written statement of the main terms and conditions of their employment should contain the items shown in Figure 6.5 and is often provided as a letter of employment. Contractual rights vary from contract to contract and only apply to the employer and employee who are parties to that contract.

A job description is a requirement in ISO 17025:1999 and ISO 15189:2002 and is a major source of information regarding a contractual relationship. A job description is best seen as separate from a person specification and the terms and conditions of employment. However, job descriptions are often produced which contain terms and conditions of employment (Figure 6.5). It is a matter of choice as to whether the job description should contain this information.

• Name and address of the employer	• Hours of work
• Place of work	• Sickness and sick pay arrangements
• Name of employee	• Holiday pay and entitlement
• Date employment begins	• Any pension scheme
• Date job will end if not permanent	• Notice period for termination of employment
• Job title	• Disciplinary and grievance arrangements
• Rate of pay and the interval between payments	• Details of collective (trade union) agreements

modified from Written Statements in the ACAS Employment Handbook, A-Z of Work (2001)

Figure 6.5 Terms and conditions of employment

FUNCTION OF JOB DESCRIPTIONS
Job descriptions play a pivotal role in personnel and quality management. Figure 6.6 indicates some of the most important functions of a job description.

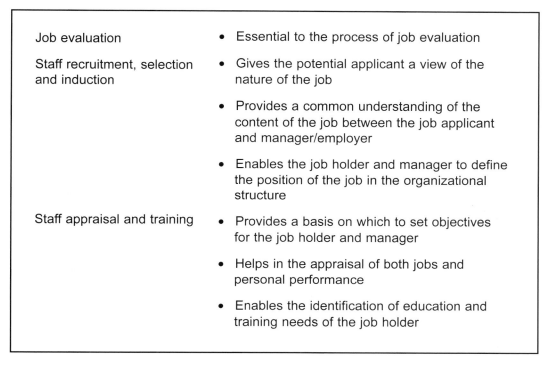

Job evaluation	• Essential to the process of job evaluation
Staff recruitment, selection and induction	• Gives the potential applicant a view of the nature of the job
	• Provides a common understanding of the content of the job between the job applicant and manager/employer
	• Enables the job holder and manager to define the position of the job in the organizational structure
Staff appraisal and training	• Provides a basis on which to set objectives for the job holder and manager
	• Helps in the appraisal of both jobs and personal performance
	• Enables the identification of education and training needs of the job holder

Figure 6.6 Functions of a job description

FORMAT AND CONTENT

At St Elsewhere's the format of job descriptions is the same throughout the laboratory and individual job descriptions are created using a form [MF-GEN-JobDesc]. Figure 6.7 gives an example for a Medical Laboratory Assistant (MLA) in Haematology. It is important that similar jobs have similar responsibilities and content. For example, if MLA's are employed in different disciplines within pathology then, although the job descriptions in each situation might vary in the detailed content, they should reflect the same levels of responsibility. If a number of different people are writing job descriptions it is important to give one individual the task of checking for format and style.

The job title should be easily understood throughout an organization and not contain any element of discrimination, for example the job title 'laboratory cleaner' should be used rather than 'cleaning lady'. The location states where in the pathology laboratory the individual is employed.

As with the person specification form, the informative file name of the job description form [MF-GEN-JobDesc] can be adjusted to create a unique filename for the record made by using the form. For example, the record filename for the

MLA in Figure 6.7 is MF-HAE-JobDesc#MLA. Some posts, such as that of Pathology Computer Manager, will require separate and distinctive job descriptions [MF-GEN-JobDesc#CompMan], but at the level of MLA in Haematology the same job description could be used for the three posts in that department.

Not many job descriptions include an organization chart, but it is probably the most satisfactory way of conveying to an individual employee their position in an organization and to whom they are accountable (Figure 6.7). The purpose of the job should be brief, concise and aim to convey to the reader the main aspects of the job. The main duties and responsibilities can be sub-divided into different areas if that makes the presentation easier to follow. The focus should be on what the job holder does rather than on how they do it. Each phrase should start with an action verb in the third person singular, present tense, such as assist, analyze, prepare, perform, report etc. General responsibilities in relation to health and safety and confidentiality are best separated from main duties and responsibilities. The paragraph, joint review and the job description introduces the idea that the review is a shared activity between the manager and the employee, and that at an annual joint review, the content of a job might change.

INDUCTION AND ORIENTATION
'Ideal Standard' clause 6.2.3 Induction and orientation

GENERAL
Staff induction is the first opportunity to orientate a new employee to the work place, and in that sense is the earliest part of staff development and training. The induction begins during recruitment and selection, but this section will focus on the first day at work onwards. What is important to any new employee, particularly to a school leaver who may have had no previous experience of the work place, is what to do on the first day. Where and when to report, who to report to, what to bring, and if arriving by car or bicycle where to park. To block the parking space reserved for the Director of Pathology would not be the ideal way to begin a new job!

The nature of the induction, who does it and when, will vary depending on the size and nature of the laboratory's host organization; it should, however, be done in a systematic way. At St Elsewhere's as the induction proceeds a record is kept using a staff induction form [MF-GEN-StafInd], and the whole process is constantly monitored to ensure that all important aspects have been dealt with. This induction checklist should be part of the employees' personnel record and provides evidence at an accreditation inspection that an induction scheme is in operation.

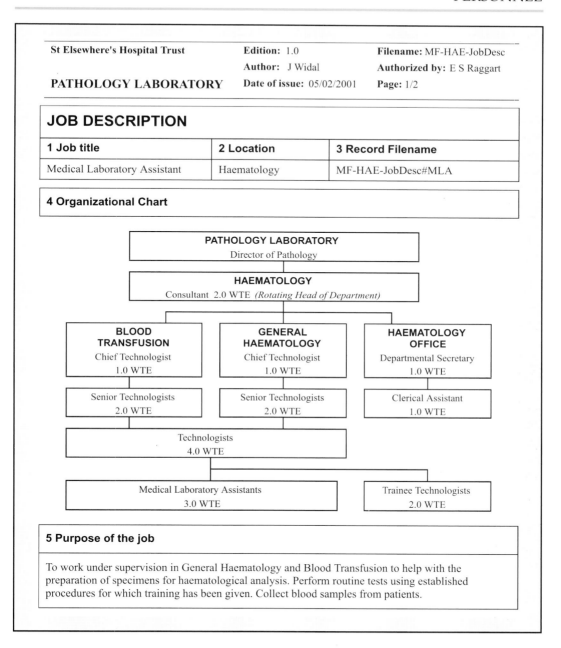

St Elsewhere's Hospital Trust | **Edition:** 1.0 | **Filename:** MF-HAE-JobDesc

Author: J Widal | **Authorized by:** E S Raggart

PATHOLOGY LABORATORY | **Date of issue:** 05/02/2001 | **Page:** 1/2

JOB DESCRIPTION

1 Job title	2 Location	3 Record Filename
Medical Laboratory Assistant	Haematology	MF-HAE-JobDesc#MLA

4 Organizational Chart

PATHOLOGY LABORATORY
Director of Pathology

HAEMATOLOGY
Consultant 2.0 WTE *(Rotating Head of Department)*

BLOOD TRANSFUSION	**GENERAL HAEMATOLOGY**	**HAEMATOLOGY OFFICE**
Chief Technologist 1.0 WTE	Chief Technologist 1.0 WTE	Departmental Secretary 1.0 WTE
Senior Technologists 2.0 WTE	Senior Technologists 2.0 WTE	Clerical Assistant 1.0 WTE

Technologists
4.0 WTE

Medical Laboratory Assistants 3.0 WTE	Trainee Technologists 2.0 WTE

5 Purpose of the job

To work under supervision in General Haematology and Blood Transfusion to help with the preparation of specimens for haematological analysis. Perform routine tests using established procedures for which training has been given. Collect blood samples from patients.

Figure 6.7 Job description for a Medical Laboratory Assistant in Haematology

St Elsewhere's Hospital Trust	**Edition:** 1.0	**Filename:** MF-HAE-JobDesc
	Author: J Widal	**Authorized by:** E S Raggart
PATHOLOGY LABORATORY	**Date of issue:** 05/02/2001	**Page:** 1/2

6 Main duties and responsibilities

All duties will be performed according to written laboratory procedures and after appropriate training by a designated supervisor.

6.1 Specimen collection, registration and preparation
- Perform venepuncture on patients.
- Sort and identify specimens received.
- Register patient details and tests required on the laboratory computer.
- Prepare samples where appropriate for analysis.

6.2 Technical duties
- Perform certain tests under supervision and keep records of test results.
- After checking by designated supervisor, enter test results on laboratory computer.
- Use and operate equipment such as centrifuges, automated equipment, pipettes and computer terminals.

6.3 General duties
- Prepare solutions and reagents.
- Clean and sterilise laboratory equipment, shelves, bench tops and sinks.
- Dispose of contaminated material including sharps.
- Undertake any other responsibility which may be reasonably allocated by designated supervisor

7 General responsibilities

- Participate in all activities which seek to ensure compliance with the 'Ideal Standard' accreditation scheme.
- Comply at all times with the Laboratory Safety Policy.
- Report/ensure that any defect which may affect safety at work is brought to the attention of the designated supervisor.
- Respect information obtained in the course of duties performed, and refrain from disclosing such information without the consent of the employee/patient, or person entitled to act on their behalf, except where disclosure is required by law or by the order of a Court, or is necessary in the public interest.

8 Job description and the annual Joint Review

This job description reflects the present requirement of the post. It will be reviewed and revised, in consultation with the job holder, as and when duties and responsibilities change. Such reviews will normally take place at the annual joint review meeting.

Job holder's signature:	John Jones	Date:	05/02/2001
Manager's signature:	J Widal	Date:	05/02/2001

Figure 6.7 continued Job description for a Medical Laboratory Assistant in Haematology

The amount of information which needs to be imparted to the new employee may well seem alarming and confusing and should, therefore, be imparted over a period of time; not too much being attempted on the first day. If the parent organization has a staff handbook this can be a useful reference source for a new employee. A number of people will be involved in the induction process and who does what could be part of the staff induction checklist. If the new employee is coming as a trainee technologist in the Haematology Department, then they might meet the Head of Department briefly and be conducted through the first day by the Chief Technologist or an assigned deputy. At St Elsewhere's, a suitable person of similar grade is assigned to befriend the new recruit in the first few weeks, showing them where the toilets are, where to eat lunch, and inviting them to join in some social activity like a visit to a bowling alley one evening.

St Elsewhere's Hospital Trust has a personnel department which holds induction courses only every two months and, therefore, a large amount of the initial work has to be done by pathology laboratory staff. Whatever the format of the induction checklist, it is important that the process imparts to new employees information categorised under headings shown in Figure 6.8.

Organizational information
- nature of the organization, its history and where the employee's department fits it

Procedural information
- terms and conditions of employment
- disciplinary and grievance procedures
- health and safety procedures
- fire and bomb procedures
- standards or codes of dress
- rules on entering and leaving the premises

Job information
- a job description including an organization chart
- details of any training
- procedures for obtaining equipment, stationery or tools

Personal information
- how salaries are paid
- location of dining room
- location of changing facilities and toilets

Team information
- information about the employee's immediate workplace
- informal information to make the individual feel part of the team

---

Figure 6.8 Categories of information for new employees

DISCIPLINARY RULES AND GRIEVANCE PROCEDURES

One area of induction that is generally poorly dealt with is information concerning disciplinary rules and procedures and grievance procedures. It is important to explain the purpose of the rules and procedures and deal with this area in an open way. In a sense they are two sides of a coin, what the employer expects of the employee and vice versa. Figure 6.9 provides definitions from the ACAS 'Code of Practice on Disciplinary and Grievance Procedures'.

Disciplinary rules and procedures are necessary for promoting orderly employment relations as well as fairness and consistency in the treatment of individuals. They enable organizations to influence the conduct of workers and deal with problems of poor performance and attendance thereby assisting organizations to operate effectively. Rules set standards of conduct and performance at work; procedures help ensure standards are adhered to and also provide a fair method of dealing with alleged failures to deal with them.

In any organization workers may have problems or concerns about their work, working environment or working relationships that they may wish to raise and have addressed. A **grievance procedure** provides a mechanism for these to be dealt with fairly and speedily, before they develop into major problems and potentially collective disputes.

based on the Code of Practice on Disciplinary and Grievance Procedures, ACAS (2000)

Figure 6.9 Disciplinary rules and grievance procedures

ANNUAL JOINT REVIEW

'Ideal Standard' clause 6.2.4 Annual joint review

A number of accreditation systems require that the organization should have some form of documented procedure in which there are regular meetings between a member of staff and their immediate supervisor. The concept appears under a number of different titles such as staff appraisal, employee appraisal, performance review or annual review. The type of procedure that is adopted by an organization will depend on the way in which the organization conducts its business.

In general there is a move away from 'staff appraisal' towards 'joint review'. The emphasis being away from 'something being done to somebody' to a review that seeks to 'examine the needs of the organization and of the individual in order to improve the quality of the service given to the users and to encourage productive working relationships'. This approach is well illustrated in Figure 6.2 from ISO 9004:2000, which emphasises the involvement of people as an essential part of making and sustaining improvements in an organization. Joint review is not only a 'once a year' activity, but in a well run organization is supplemented by frequent informal contact between the immediate supervisor and the staff member. A word of praise or a timely piece of cautionary advice is just as valuable as the formal review. No one scheme is ideal, but what is important is that the benefits shown in Figure 6.10 are realised by all parties.

Benefits to the job holder

- Opportunity to discuss all aspects of the job, with the boss, in depth and away from pressures of daily workload.

- Clarifies how to contribute to the objectives of the department, and the aims of the organization.

- Identifies strengths and weaknesses, building on the former and addressing the latter.

- Gives clear direction as to what is expected in the job, involving the holder in planning their work and their future.

- Recording the interview and action plan signifies a mutual commitment.

Benefits to the boss

- Creates an opportunity for managers to think seriously about what they expect of their staff and clarifies plans for the future.

- Opportunity to recognise new ideas and tackle problem areas.

- Clarifies and improves relationships between the two parties, and strengthens the role of the manager as a leader.

Benefits to the organization

- Appraisal represents a visible commitment by an organization to the importance of its staff.

- Creates an opportunity for greater individual effectiveness and commitment to corporate aims.

Figure 6.10 Benefits of an annual joint review

This process of annual joint review is the first example in this book of a 'cycle of continual improvement'. An approach to quality improvement used in the Pathology Laboratory at St Elsewhere's Hospital (see Chapter 11, Figure 11.17). This is illustrated in Figure 6.11 which shows the inter-connectivity of the clauses of the 'Ideal Standard' involved.

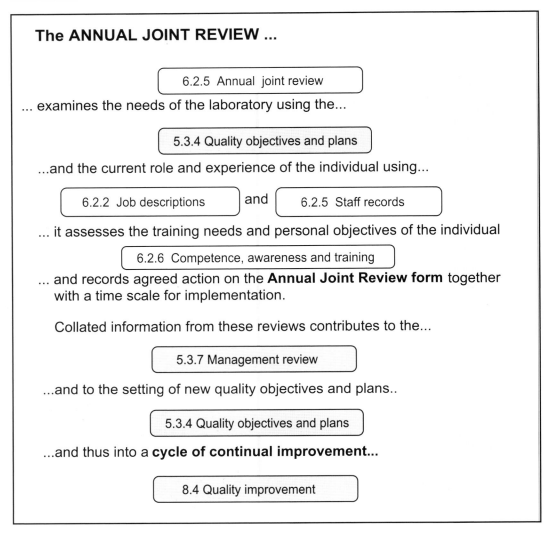

The ANNUAL JOINT REVIEW ...

6.2.5 Annual joint review

... examines the needs of the laboratory using the...

5.3.4 Quality objectives and plans

...and the current role and experience of the individual using...

6.2.2 Job descriptions   and   6.2.5 Staff records

... it assesses the training needs and personal objectives of the individual

6.2.6 Competence, awareness and training

... and records agreed action on the **Annual Joint Review form** together with a time scale for implementation.

Collated information from these reviews contributes to the...

5.3.7 Management review

...and to the setting of new quality objectives and plans..

5.3.4 Quality objectives and plans

...and thus into a **cycle of continual improvement...**

8.4 Quality improvement

Figure 6.11 Annual joint review – a cycle of continual improvement

The approach to the annual joint review adopted at St Elsewhere's, and the form used is shown in Figure 6.12. It is essential that a generous, but defined amount of time, free of interruptions is allowed for the annual joint review. All reviewers should have training and be formally assessed for competence by having trial reviews in the presence of a more senior member of staff as observer.

ANNUAL JOINT REVIEW FORM

RECORD FILENAME	

1 Staff member	2 Post held	3 Location

4 Reviewer	5 Post held	6 Location

7 Date of review

8 Introduction

The purpose of this Review is to enable you and your immediate manager to take stock of how things are going for you at work - in your overall job and specific work plans, in your working relationships with other people, and any other aspects of working in Pathology.

In short, Joint Reviews - taking place throughout the Hospital Trust - are designed to

'examine the needs of the organization and of the individual in order to improve the quality of the service given to the users and to encourage productive working relationships within the Trust'

Most jobs and people are developing all the time. It is therefore likely that out of the Review will emerge some points for action - by you, your manager, and/or others - to help you and your work develop further during the next year.

This form and the current objectives for the Pathology Laboratory (attached) are provided to help you and your manager obtain maximum benefit from the Review. Topics have been laid out to provide some talking points - but this should not prevent discussion about other aspects of your working life. Please prepare for the Review by going through the papers. A set of these papers is also being sent to your manager who will prepare thoughts for your review.

At the end of your Review, agreed action points should be completed. These notes are for your benefit as well as your manager and will be available to your manager's manager if required. The other working papers will remain in the possession of you and your manager unless you both wish and agree otherwise.

If you have any queries at all about the Annual Joint Review, do please get in touch with the Human Resources Department.

Figure 6.12 Annual joint review form

9 Preparation

9.1. The job

a) What are the main tasks or responsibilities in your job?
(Please refer to the job description and note any major changes over the last year)

b) Which areas of your work do you think have gone particularly well during the past year?
(Please say why you think this is)

c) Which areas of your work have proved most difficult during the past year?
(Please say why you think this is)

d) How would you anticipate your job could develop or otherwise change·over the next year?
(Please note any items which you feel should be given priority attention)

9.2 Working Relationships

a) Who are your main work contacts? (Please indicate where other people most directly affect, or are affected by, the way you perform your job)
    i) The ones who most directly affect the way I perform my job are:
    ii) The ones who are most affected by the way I perform my job are:

b) What support and assistance with work do you receive from and give to others?
(Please note instances where this works particularly well or less well.)
        i) Support and assistance received from others:
        ii) Support and assistance given to others:

c) How would you like to see your working relationships change or develop over the next year?

9.3 The Department and You

a) How do you feel in general terms about working in your department? (Please indicate anything you feel particularly happy or unhappy about in your department and its work)

b) How do you see your future within your department?
(Please indicate any particular aspirations and ambitions you have)

9.4 Other aspects

Are there any other points you would like to raise that have not been covered so far?
(Please attach additional sheets as required)

9.5 Ideas for Action (Joint and individual)

a) What would you like to see done to help with things indicated above (in Sections 9.1-9.4)?

b) What could you do to help things along?

10 Agreed action

Signature of staff member		Signature of reviewer	

Item	Agreed objective	Agreed action	Timescale	Resources required	Criteria for success
1.					
2.					

Figure 6.12 continued Annual joint review form

Section 10 of the form records agreed action and is normally a separate page presented in landscape. A number of professional bodies have developed approaches to the creation of this record. The Institute of Biomedical Sciences (UK), in response to an initiative of the NHS Executive (UK) have developed an approach to personal development plans for its members and managers. Section 10 in Figure 6.12 is partly modelled on this material and action points are made in a manner that aims to be **s**pecific, **m**easurable, **a**greed, **r**ealistic and **t**imed (**smart**). Figure 6.13 shows some agreed action for the joint review of Elizabeth Rate, a trainee technologist in Haematology.

10 Agreed action					
Signature of staff member	Elizabeth Rate	**Signature of reviewer**		Margaret Jones	
Item	**Agreed objective**	**Agreed action**	**Timescale**	**Resources required**	**Criteria for success**
1.	More experience of automated ESR's [LP-HAE-AutoESR]	M Jones to arrange practical training with B Rubin	3 months	Time-one day B Rubin	Examination audit of [LP-HAE-AutoESR]
2.	Use of Microsoft Word procedure templates	Practical instruction from M Jones	3 months	3 hours with M Jones	Evidence of completion
3.	Practical experience of writing procedures	M Jones to set 3 practical tasks	6 months	As required with M Jones	Completion of practical tasks
4.	Improve participation in Departmental projects	M Jones to arrange place on course	1 year	Trust course, PR 07/ 5days plus debrief with M Jones	Certificate of successful participation

Figure 6.13 Annual joint review – agreed action points

STAFF RECORDS

'Ideal Standard' clause 6.2.5 Staff records

Staff records are an important part of any organization; they provide the basic information for human resource policies, plans and procedures. If the organization is large, then it is likely to have a personnel department that will either keep staff records within the department or at least require that records in the pathology laboratory are kept to a certain standard and format. ISO 15189:2002 requires laboratory management to maintain records of relevant educational and professional qualifications, training and experience and competence of all personnel. Good practice in personnel management suggests more extensive records should be kept and the items required are indicated in Figure 6.14.

Personal details	• name/sex/date of birth/address
	• education/qualifications
	• tax code/insurance number
	• next of kin
	• name, address and telephone number of doctor
	• details of any disability
	• professional registration
Employment details	• record of posts held with dates, job titles and salary progression
Job description	• copy of current job description
Terms and conditions of employment	• (see Figure 6.5 for further information)
Staff induction checklist	• (see Figure 6.8 for further information)
Training record	• date and details of internal and external courses and conferences attended
Joint review records	• (see Figures 6.12 and 6.13 for further information)
Occupational health record (may be held in occupational health department)	• immunisations • eyesight checks etc.
Absence record	• sickness • lateness (authorized/unauthorized)
Accident record	•
Record of disciplinary action	• (see Figure 6.9 for further information)
Correspondence	•

Figure 6.14 The staff record

COMPETENCE, AWARENESS AND TRAINING
'Ideal Standard' clause 6.2.6 Competence, awareness and training

COMPETENCE
As we have seen in Chapter 3, although the word 'competence' appears in the title of both the laboratory standards ISO 17025:1999 and ISO 15189:2002, it is not formally defined in either document. Chapter 4 discussed the concept of the competence of an organization in terms of ethical behaviour and in this chapter it is examined in terms of the competence of individuals. In ISO/DIS 19011:2002 'Guidelines on the quality and/or environmental management systems', competence is defined as 'demonstrated ability to apply knowledge and skills'. This implies that in addition to a person having the ability to apply knowledge and skills to a particular task, there must be some objective test to substantiate this ability and this is discussed later in this chapter.

COMPETENCE REQUIREMENTS
Specific competencies required to undertake a particular role or task will vary in relation to the nature of the role or task. In relation to the laboratory director (including the head of a discipline/department in pathology), ISO 15189:2002 requires 'the laboratory to be directed by a person or persons with executive responsibility who have the competence to assume responsibility for the services provided'. The notes to this clause define competence as 'the product of basic academic, postgraduate, and continuing education, as well as training and experience of several years in a medical laboratory' and say that the person or persons referred to are designated collectively as 'laboratory director'. In the context of St Elsewhere's this would mean the Director of Pathology, heads of department and nominated deputies. There is an implied assumption that competence referred to is a 'demonstrated' competence. In all fields of healthcare there is not only increasing interest in methods of demonstrating competence, but also in the maintenance of competence through the continuing professional development and revalidation of the individual.

In ISO 15189:2002 there are a number of requirements regarding the competencies necessary to fulfil the role of a laboratory director, but little attention is paid to competencies required by other groups of staff. ISO 15189:2002 requires that the responsibilities of the laboratory director shall include 'professional, scientific, consultative or advisory, organizational, administrative and educational matters' that are relevant to the services offered by the laboratory. These responsibilities, reordered to fit with the structure of the 'Ideal Standard', are shown in Figure 6.15.

4 Quality management system

- Implement the quality management system. The laboratory director and professional laboratory personnel should participate as members of the various quality improvement committees of the institution, if applicable.

5 Organization and management responsibility

- Serve as an active member of the medical staff for those facilities served, if applicable and appropriate.
- Relate to and function effectively with applicable accrediting and regulating agencies, administrative officials, the healthcare community and the patient population served.
- Plan and set goals, and develop and allocate resources appropriate to the medical environment.
- Provide effective and efficient administration of the medical laboratory service, including budget planning and control with responsible financial management, in accordance with institutional assignment of such responsibilities.

6 Resource management

- Ensure that there are sufficient qualified personnel with adequate documented training and experience to meet the needs of the laboratory.
- Provide educational programmes for the medical and laboratory staff, participate in education programmes of the institution.
- Implement a safe laboratory environment in compliance with good practice and applicable regulations.
- Ensure good staff morale.

7 Examination processes

- Provide advice to requestors about the choice of tests, the use of the laboratory services and the interpretation of laboratory data.
- Correlate laboratory data for diagnosis and patient management.
- Plan and direct research and development appropriate to the facility.
- Select and monitor all referral laboratories for quality of service.

8 Evaluation and quality improvement

- Define, implement and monitor standards of performance and quality improvement of the medical laboratory services.
- Monitor all work performed in the laboratory to determine that medically reliable data are being produced.
- Address any complaint, request or suggestion from users of the laboratory service.

Figure 6.15 Responsibilities of a laboratory director

So far the discussion has focused on professional, scientific and technical competencies, but in all jobs there will be a need for interpersonal skills. Some of these are expressed in relation to colleagues and patients in 'Good Medical Practice in Pathology' (published by The Royal College of Pathologists in the UK) that sets out a code of professional conduct for doctors registered to practice pathology. Although there are variations between disciplines, some primary elements are illustrated in Figure 6.16. In the introduction the President of the College under-lines the document's importance by saying 'Since they represent a code of prac-tice by which you will eventually be judged in terms of annual appraisal and revalidation, it is important that you are aware of the contents...'

To maintain good standards of laboratory and clinical practice by:
- keeping your professional skills and knowledge up-to-date
- ensuring that your professional beliefs do not prejudice the provision of, or access to, diagnostic or clinical services
- being honest and trustworthy
- respecting patient confidentiality
- recognising the limits of personal professional competence
- working with colleagues in ways that best serve patient's interests
- acting quickly to protect patients from risk if there is good reason to believe that a diagnostic or clinical service is performing inadequately or that you or a colleague may not be fit to practice

To maintain good standards of laboratory practice by:
- providing clinicians with information on the scope and range of laboratory services
- maintaining the highest standards of laboratory service
- maintaining the highest standards of analytical provision

To maintain good standards of clinical practice by:
- making the care of your patient your first concern
- treating every patient politely and considerately
- respecting patients' dignity and privacy
- listening to patients and respecting their views
- giving patients information in a way they can understand
- respecting the rights of patients to be fully involved in decisions about their care

from 'The duties of a doctor registered to practice chemical pathology' in 'Guidelines on Good Medical Practice in Pathology', The Royal College of Pathologists 2001

Figure 6.16 Good standards of laboratory and clinical practice

In recent years there have been major failures in the provision of pathology serv-ices and deficiencies identified in the performance of senior staff. Participation in continuing professional development programmes and revalidation of compe-tence is likely to become increasingly mandatory in the face of public concern. Under its Royal Charter, the Royal College of Pathologists in the UK, has the responsibility of maintaining professional standards in pathology practice. A recent publication, 'Sub-standard professional performance: guidance for Trusts and pathologists', outlines its approach to investigation of sub-standard perform-ance. A performance review approach is detailed that combines thorough investi-gation with support for pathologists under investigation or suspension and emphasises the importance of retraining where indicated. The aims of retraining are to facilitate the restoration of professional skills, the restoration of an individual's professional and personal self-confidence and reinforcement of high professional standards. This approach to retraining could be equally applicable to any professional group within pathology.

EVIDENCE OF COMPETENCE
Evidence of competence can be demonstrated in a number of ways, professional registration and revalidation certificates, records of courses attended and continuing professional development points attained and training records kept by the individual staff member and the laboratory. The development of statutory registers is often preceeded by professionals creating a voluntary register, such as the recently developed, European Register for Clinical Chemists.

AWARENESS AND TRAINING
To be aware in the context of the medical laboratory can be defined as 'having knowledge and being informed of current developments'. This state of awareness is achieved both by training, (bringing people to an agreed standard of proficiency) and by continuing education (continuing to acquire knowledge).

Figure 6.2 identifies the need for an organization to encourage the development of its staff by 'providing ongoing training and career planning'. The process of the annual joint review described earlier (Figure 6.12) will define the training and continuing education needs of individuals in the context of a laboratory's quality objectives and plans. It also records a joint commitment by the employer and the employee.

In different countries there are different arrangements for training staff. The content of the training will also depend upon the level of entry of the staff member and their role in the organization. Some new employees will come to their post fully qualified having undertaken their education and training in other organizations, but for some it will be their first job. For the former, a familiarization programme at induction may be all that is required, but for the new entrant a documented training scheme will be very important. In many professions, postgraduate training is undertaken only in institutions that are accredited for training purposes. The professional bodies which represent these professions will have a system of monitoring the institutions providing the training and will provide training log books as well as visiting the trainees at regular intervals to ensure that they are being provided with the appropriate opportunities to gain experience and training.

As the purpose of any training programme is to ensure the competence to undertake a particular role (e.g. that of a Health and Safety Officer), or a task, such as analysing patient samples for lithium content. It is essential that training records are kept and that there is evidence of competence. This chapter deals with training records and Chapter 11 discusses the role of the witness audit in providing evidence of competence. Figure 6.17 illustrates a partially completed training record [MF-BIO-TrnRec#John Startup] for John Startup, a trainee technologist in Biochemistry. This basic design can be adapted for any situation by entering the filename and name of any procedure in the left hand side columns. Completion with the trainers signature indicates an assessment of competence, which may be by the conduct of an examination audit or by verbal interrogation depending on the particular procedure being assessed.

St Elsewhere's Hospital Trust	Edition: 1.0	Filename: MP-GEN-TrnRec
	Author: J. Qualiman	Authorized by: W.Jaggard
PATHOLOGY LABORATORY	Date of issue: 05/02/2000	Page: 1/3

TRAINING RECORD

RECORD FILENAME	MF-BIO-TrnRec#John Startup

1 Name	2 Post held	3 Location
John Startup	Trainee Technologist	Biochemistry
4 Date employment commenced	**5 Date employment finished**	**6 Co-ordinating supervisor**
03/01/2001		Alfred Johnson

Course or Procedure filename/version	Procedure name	Date training started	Date training completed	Trainee's signature	Trainer's signature
Elementary First Aid certificate	-	12/11/2000	12/11/2000	J Startup	J Solom
LP-GEN-SpecRec / v 1.1	Specimen reception	08/01/2001	12/01/2001	J Startup	Al Johnson
LP-BIO-SpecRef / v 2.1	Specimen referral	08/01/2001	12/01/2001	J Startup	Al Johnson
LP-BIO-BldGas / v 1.1	Blood Gas Analyzer	15/01/2001	19/01/2001	J Startup	Al Johnson
LP-BIO-SerumLi / v 1.2	Serum Lithium	15/01/2001	25/01/2001	J Startup	Al Johnson
LP-BIO-ABCAnal / v 1.1	ABC Analyzer	26/01/2001			

Figure 6.17 Partially completed training record [MF-BIO-TrnRec#John Startup]

As can be seen from Figure 6.17, training courses can also be included in such a record. In products such as Q-Pulse these training records can be created automatically and when a new version of a procedure or a new procedure is introduced this can automatically be posted to the training record as a new requirement for training or re-training for that individual.

CONTINUING EDUCATION

There is always a need for continuing education and training in an organization such as a Pathology Laboratory. The form it will take depends on the needs of the individual and of the bodies which increasingly regulate the continuing education, revalidation and accreditation of individuals. Monitoring the need for continuing education can usefully take place at the annual joint review. It is important that all staff have ready access to library and information services and a quiet place in which to study. Resources must be available to allow staff to attend appropriate meetings.

THE WORLD WIDE WEB

The advent of the world wide web has vastly increased ready access to information for training and continuing education. Free access to this resource and training in using it effectively are twin requisites for any laboratory. Its use for e-mail and discussion groups is of enormous value. However, in dealing with the surfeit of information available, it is important to assess to what extent the information available in certain areas has been validated. There are many texts written about the use of the Internet but the author has found using the search engine 'Google' www.google.com to be the most effective way to start.

MEETINGS AND COMMUNICATION
'Ideal Standard' clause 6.2.7 Meetings and communication

MEETINGS

Meetings take place at different levels in any organization. In St Elsewhere's the direct line of reporting is from departmental management meetings to the Pathology Management Board, and from pathology management to the Directorate of Diagnostic and Therapeutic Medicine and thence to the Management Board of the hospital. Meetings at these levels are conducted in a formal manner and minutes are kept (Figure 5.20). Open staff meetings for the whole of pathology and in individual departments are also held on a regular basis (bimonthly) that are less formal and notes are taken. These meetings are a very important opportunity for a wider group of staff to participate in the functioning of the laboratory, and for management to learn at first hand the concerns of the staff.

COMMUNICATION AND INFORMATION SHARING

Information sharing needs an understanding of what information should be shared and the mechanisms for sharing. In any organization there is always an informal 'grapevine' through which information or misinformation will travel. In the case of misinformation this can often cause unnecessary distress and concern. If systems are in place for information sharing then the information passing through the system must be reliable and clearly presented. The Management Board of St Elsewhere's produce a report of the annual management review (Figure 11.21) that includes a section on future quality objectives. The aim is to give staff a better understanding of how they might organize their personal objectives. Briefing notes, produced at regular intervals and either sent to selected individuals for onward dissemination or displayed prominently throughout the organization, assist in the process of communication. However, it is crucial that information should not just come down through an organization, but should also travel upwards, either through the medium of minutes of meetings, through feedback during verbal briefings, or other methods such as staff suggestions, audits and through monitoring complaints.

Chapter 7

Premises, health, safety and welfare

INTRODUCTION
'Ideal Standard' clauses 6.3 Premises / 6.6 Health, safety and welfare
This chapter looks at two closely inter-related issues, firstly, laboratory premises and the work environment and secondly, arrangements for the health, safety and welfare of any personnel or users who have cause to be within the laboratory, or who might be affected by the functioning of the laboratory. In ISO 9001:2000, clause 6.3 'Infrastructure', refers to buildings, workspace and associated utilities, process equipment and supporting services. In ISO 17025:1999 and ISO 15189:2002 clauses 5.3 and 5.2 are entitled, 'Accommodation and environmental conditions'. The committee draft of a newly emerging standard ISO 15190 deals with safety management in the medical laboratory. This chapter focuses on the buildings and workspace, and Chapter 8 on equipment and supporting services.

The emphasis in ISO 17025:1999 is on facilitating 'the correct performance of the tests' and on monitoring environmental conditions where they might 'influence the quality of results'. As would perhaps be expected in a standard for medical laboratories, ISO 15189:2002 extends these requirements to a concern that the laboratory is designed not only, for 'the efficiency of its operation', but also, 'that consideration be given to the comfort of its occupants' and that 'the risk of injury and occupational illness is minimised'. This additional emphasis is also a requirement in CPA(UK)Ltd and NPAAC standards.

Different quality and accreditation systems may stress different requirements for facilities, premises and equipment, and for the health, safety and welfare of staff. However, irrespective of the requirements of international standards, individual countries will have legislation (regulations, codes of practice and guidelines) which set standards for the workplace, whether it is a factory, an office block or a pathology laboratory. To illustrate these legislative approaches, reference is made in this chapter under health, safety and welfare to relevant Directives promulgated within the European Community (EC). These Directives not only establish the standards required, but also represent a practical approach to the management of premises and equipment, and to ensuring the health, safety and welfare of all persons likely to be affected by the functioning of a pathology laboratory.

Figure 7.1 illustrates the inter-connectivity between the clauses and sub-clauses of the 'Ideal standard' that relate to premises and the working environment and to health, safety and welfare.

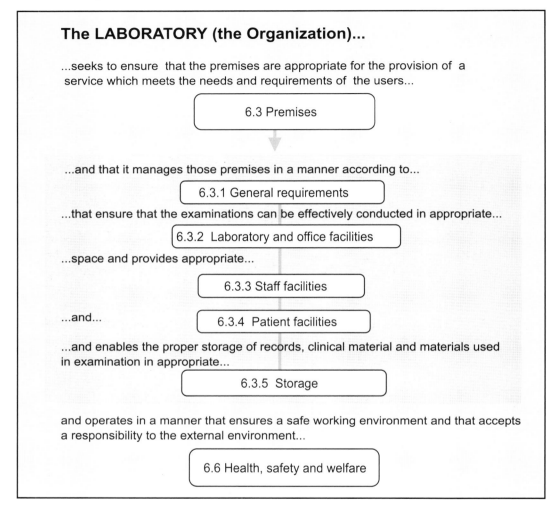

Figure 7.1 Clauses 6.3 and 6.6 of the 'Ideal Standard' – Premises / Health, safety and welfare

GENERAL REQUIREMENTS
'Ideal Standard' clause 6.3.1 General requirements
The nature and extent of the premises which constitute the pathology laboratory in a hospital are determined by three main factors:

- the services which are offered, e.g. are clinics or phlebotomy services provided within the laboratory area?, are blood products available on a 24 hour basis from the laboratory?

- the tests offered, e.g. are radioisotopes used or are pathogenic organisms isolated and cultured?

- are staff facilities, such as rest rooms or seminar/library facilities, available within the laboratory area or conveniently nearby?

Depending on their scope and purpose, pathology laboratories will have a variety of facilities and activities and Figure 7.2 summarises the main requirements of ISO 15189:2002. It can be seen from this figure that the physical facilities and concept of a pathology laboratory are much more than the area in which examination (analytical) processes are conducted.

The laboratory shall have arrangements to ensure...

- adequate space for the workload undertaken, designed and environmentally controlled in a manner that does not compromise the quality of the work or the service to users (including sites remote from the main laboratory)

- effective separation of incompatible activities

- controlled access to areas where examinations are conducted and samples and confidential records are kept

- appropriate communications

- the health, safety and welfare of laboratory staff

- the protection of patients and visitors from known hazards

- the privacy and comfort of patients

- appropriate storage space for quality and process records, clinical material and materials used in the course of examinations

based on ISO 15189:2002 clause 5.2 'Accommodation and environmental conditions'

Figure 7.2 ISO 15189:2002 clause 5.2 – Accommodation and environmental conditions

LABORATORY AND OFFICE FACILITIES

'Ideal Standard' clause 6.3.2 Laboratory and office facilities

The first item in Figure 7.2 introduces the concept of 'adequate space' and has echoes from the discussion in Chapter 6 concerning 'appropriate numbers of staff'. As with staffing, assessment of adequate space will be determined by reference to any local guidelines and by professional judgement combined with objective evidence that the space provided makes it possible to give a service that meets the needs and requirements of the users. Flexibility in design is essential to accommodating changing work practices and types of equipment.

An important publication by the Health and Safety Executive (UK), 'Workplace, Health, Safety and Welfare – a short guide for managers', summarises minimum requirements for health and safety in relation to the physical aspects of premises (Figure 7.3). Some are important not only to the health and safety of staff, but also to the proper functioning of equipment or test systems.

Safety	Health
• Maintenance	• Ventilation
• Floor and traffic routes	• Temperature in indoor workplaces
• Falls and falling objects	• Lighting
• Transparent or translucent doors, gates or walls and windows	• Cleanliness and waste materials
	• Room dimensions and space
• Openable windows and the ability to clean them safely	• Workstations and seating
• Doors and gates	
• Escalators and moving walkways	

based on 'Workplace Health, Safety and Welfare – a short guide for managers' Health and Safety Executive, UK 1997

Figure 7.3   Physical aspects of premises in relation to health and safety

In each category there are issues to be considered when assessing or designing a workplace e.g. Does the workplace have enough free space to allow people to move around with ease? Later in this chapter an approach to converting these minimum requirements into a practical 'good housekeeping' audit checklist will be discussed.

The second item raised in Figure 7.2 is the 'effective separation of incompatible activities' and ISO 15189:2002 provides some specific and familiar examples for consideration (Figure 7.4).

Separation of activities is required where...

- examination procedures pose a hazard (e.g. mycobacteriology, radionuclides)

- the work may be affected or influenced by not being separated (e.g. nucleic acid amplifications)

- an environment conducive to quiet and uninterrupted work is required (e.g. cytopathology screening)

- work requires a controlled environment (e.g. large computer systems)

based on ISO 15189:2002 'Medical laboratories – Particular requirements for quality and competence'

Figure 7.4 Separation of incompatible activities

One such need for separation is emphasised in the recently updated NHS Estates (UK) publication, 'Facilities for the mortuary and postmortem room services'. The facilities are described as 'fulfilling five functions, which, as far as possible, should be kept physically separate'; the receipt and temporary storage of bodies, investigations into the cause of death by performing a PM of the body, the demonstration of PM findings in cases of clinical interest or for teaching purposes, the viewing/identification of a body and accommodating visiting relatives/next of kin. This design and briefing document provides 'schedules of accommodation' and 'modular approach to planning' that enables those preparing plans for refurbishment or new build of facilities to pick and mix what is required. As a response to serious situations in which the dignity of the deceased has not been adequately respected, simple but valuable advice is provided on planning temporary body storage facilities to cope with expected increases in deaths due to seasonal variation, the consequences of a major disaster or due to refurbishment of existing facilities.

The third point in Figure 7.2 concerns 'controlled access to areas where examinations are conducted and samples and confidential records are kept'. When a new facility is being planned, areas for public access can be separated from areas accessed by laboratory staff. However, careful thought should be given to access by other hospital personnel – porters, nurses, doctors bringing samples or collecting blood – primarily in terms of their safety. Controlled access can take the form of swipe cards or key pads, remembering that in the latter case 'reading over the shoulder' can potentially result in subsequent unauthorized access.

The subject of laboratory planning and design would be a topic for a separate publication but some 'Practical Lessons in Laboratory Planning' have been enunciated in a brief publication by a practising architect with ten years of experience working as a certified medical technologist in the USA. The five key recommendations in brief are:

1) *Involve the laboratory staff*, and by this is meant not just laboratory administrators etc, but 'people who work at the laboratory bench'.

2) *Prepare a comprehensive equipment list*, that includes dimensions, weight and the utilities and environmental requirements for the equipment. From this information the design and relationships of workstations can be developed and the need for ancillary space such as gas storage determined.

3) *Ensure that all the variables are included in area calculations.* Factor in all equipment space requirements including access for maintenance (back and front!) and requirements for storage of associated consumables and reagents. Include all safety requirements including egress codes (escape routes), and all workstation spaces, allowing space for small but often overlooked items such as pH meters, rockers and balances.

4) *Determine the relationships among your laboratory departments and all support spaces.* What can be usefully combined, what needs to separated, (incompatible activities). Insist that staff participate in the necessary iterative process as the relationship and layout diagrams are developed.

5) *Actively participate in the formulation of the bottom line.* When adjustments are made to projected costs be aware that anything added or subtracted has an associated cost and if costs have to be trimmed involve the laboratory staff in prioritising needs.

The NCCLS sub-committee for laboratory design, of which the author of the above article is a member, has prepared a guideline, GP18-A, on Laboratory Design; that 'provides a foundation of information about design elements that can be used to help define the issues being considered when designing a laboratory'. For detailed requirements for particular sections of the laboratory the College of American Pathologists, Laboratory Accreditation Program Checklists (www.cap.org) and the NPAAC, Laboratory Assessment Checklists (www.health.gov.au/npaac) are an invaluable source of information. The remaining items in Figure 7.2 are dealt with in subsequent sections of this chapter.

STAFF FACILITIES
'Ideal Standard' clause 6.3.3 Staff facilities
The provision of staff facilities has two aspects, those facilities associated with welfare, and those associated with education and training; the latter having been dealt with in Chapter 6.

CPA(UK)Ltd in Standard C2, 'Facilities for staff', (Figure 7.5) demonstrates its commitment to the welfare of staff in terms of personal safety, comfort and hygiene.

C2 Facilities for staff

All staff need facilities, within the department, to ensure personal safety, comfort and hygeine

C2.1   The premises shall have staff facilities that are readily accesible and include:

  a) sufficient toilet accomodation

  b) shower facilities where required

  c) a rest area

  d) basic catering facilities and access to a supply of drinking water

  e) a changing area and secure storage for personal effects

  f)   storage for protective clothing

  g) safe and secure working arrangements

C2.2   There shall be overnight accommodation, when neccesary, that is conveniently sited and secure.

CPA(UK)Ltd Standards for the Medical Laboratory 2001

Figure 7.5 CPA(UK)Ltd Standard C2 – Facilities for staff

The HSE publication, 'Workplace, Health, Safety and Welfare – a short guide for managers' also provides minimum requirements for welfare in premises. With respect to the welfare of staff, the regulations require the provision of sanitary conveniences and washing facilities, drinking water, accommodation for clothing and facilities for changing, and facilities for rest and to eat meals. Of particular interest in relation to staff welfare in laboratories are the standards in relation to the 'accommodation for clothing and facilities for changing' and the 'facilities for rest and to eat meals' (Figure 7.6).

Accommodation for clothing and facilities for changing

- Adequate, suitable and secure space should be provided to store workers' own clothing and special clothing. As far as is reasonably practicable the facilities should allow for drying clothing.

- Changing facilities should also be provided for workers who change into special work clothing. The facilities should be readily accesible from workrooms and washing and eating facilities and should ensure the privacy of the user.

Facilities for rest and to eat meals

- Suitable and sufficient, readily accesible, rest facilities should be provided. Rest areas or rooms should be large enough, and have sufficient seats with backrests and tables, for the number of workers likely to use them at any time. They should Include suitable facilities to eat meals where meals are regularly eaten in the workplace and the food would otherwise be likely to become contaminated.

- Seats should be provided for workers to use during breaks. These should be in a place where personal protective clothing need not be worn. Work areas can be counted as rest areas and as eating facilities, provided they are adequately clean and there is a suitable surface on which to place food. Where provided, eating facilities should include a facility for preparing or obtaining a hot drink. Where hot food cannot be obtained in, or reasonably near to, the workplace, workers may need to be provided with a means for heating their own food.

- Canteens or restaurants may be used as rest facilities provided there is no obligation to purchase food.

- Suitable rest facilities should be provided for pregnant women or nursing mothers. They should be near to sanitary facilities and, where necessary, include the facility to lie down.

- Rest areas and rest rooms away from the workstation should include suitable arrangements to protect non-smokers from discomfort caused by tobacco smoke.

based on 'Workplace, Health, Safety and Welfare - a short guide for managers'
Health and Safety Executive UK 1997

Figure 7.6   Staff accommodation requirements

PATIENT FACILITIES
'Ideal Standard' clause 6.3.4 Patient facilities

With respect to patient's facilities, two questions need to be asked. Firstly, 'What facilities should be provided?, and secondly, but often overlooked, 'How do you find them?'. With regard to what should be provided, Figure 7.7 summarises the valuable advice given in the Premises and Equipment sections of 'Guidelines for Approved Pathology Collection Centres', published by the NPAAC.

Premises and equipment should include...

- adequately lit and clean environment and a temperature controlled collection environment

- space appropriate for patient throughput

- hand washing facilities conveniently available to the collection staff

- adequate toilet facilities available for patients, staff and accompanying persons in, or conveniently adjacent to, the collection centre

- reasonable provision for the entry of ill and disabled patients

- provision for privacy during collections and adequate accommodation of appropriate accompanying persons (e.g. interpreter, guardian) during the collection

- a reception and waiting area separate from the collection area

- telephone access within the collection area

- flat surfaces available for clerical work separate from surfaces for specimen handling

- a display of the hours of operation

- suitable collection chair and/or couch for patients

- suitable storage for supplies

- basic first aid material in sites where simple procedures (e.g. phlebotomy) are performed

- equipment for resuscitation in sites where more complicated procedures are performed

based on NPAAC 'Guidelines for Approved Pathology Collection Centres' 2000

Figure 7.7 Patient facilities – guidance for premises and equipment

However, there is little point in having good facilities for patients if they are difficult to find. In conjunction with a hospital project team, the laboratory at St Elsewhere's is currently implementing the advice provided in an NHS Estates publication with the unfamiliar title of 'Wayfinding', best translated as 'finding your way'!

It usefully divides the information required by the patient or accompanying person into four categories; pre-visit information, getting to the site, getting around the site and arriving at the destination. Figure 7.8 is based upon this publication. Items marked with an asterisk are those the laboratory might provide or have an influence upon. The provision of this information will be discussed in Chapter 9 under 'Information for patients and users'. The concept 'environmental information' embraces the features of the environment that impact on the person making the journey to the laboratory. Examples would be the appearance of buildings and building entrances, prominent internal and external landmarks, 'follow the yellow line' for pathology etc. In the author's experience, quite small inexpensive adjustments to environmental information could have a major impact. At St Elsewhere's a written complaint was received from a patient who said "after following signs for blood collection and arriving at the haematology department, I found a notice on a glass panelled door saying 'no unauthorized persons beyond this point', when the reception area is clearly visible through the door". All laboratory staff should undertake these journeys pretending to be their own grandmothers!

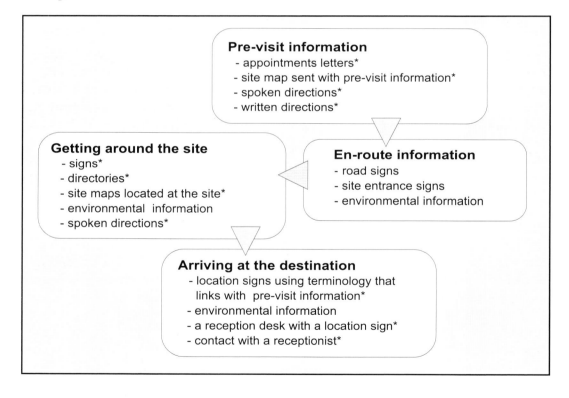

Figure 7.8 Information for visiting the laboratory

STORAGE
'Ideal Standard' clause 6.3.5 Storage

GENERAL
ISO 15189:2002 states that 'relevant storage space and conditions shall be provided to ensure the continuing integrity of samples, slides, histology blocks, retained microorganisms, document files, manuals, equipment, reagents, laboratory supplies, records and results'. This list re-emphasises the need for adequate storage for 'control of records' (Chapter 5), 'control of clinical material' (Chapter 9) and 'equipment, reagents and laboratory supplies' (Chapter 8). The inadequacy of storage space in laboratories is one of the major causes of failure in 'good housekeeping' and underlies a potential for serious incidents. In Figure 7.3, attention is draw to the dangers of falling objects and the guidance states 'materials and objects need to be stored and stacked in such a way that they are not likely to fall and cause injury'. How many high shelves are there in laboratories throughout the world on which there are 'materials and objects', kept because they might come in useful sometime! A useful question to ask is, 'if you have not used it for two years, do you need it?'.

Even with the increasing use of electronic data records a properly organized room in which documents can be systematically stored is an essential part of an effective quality management system. Storage of clinical material in an appropriate environment increases the likelihood of being able to reconstruct an examination process and reinforces 'acceptable standards of staff conduct towards human samples, tissues or remains' (Figure 4.3). It may be necessary to store records and clinical material 'offsite', in which case special care should be taken to ensure proper conditions for storage and effective mechanisms for retrieval through proper indexing.

STORAGE OF BLOOD AND BLOOD PRODUCTS
The storage of blood and blood products (and other materials used 'in vivo') represent a special case of storage governed by the nature of the material and by the fact that they are to be used 'in vivo'. Section 3, 'Preservation of blood and blood products' of the NPAAC 'Laboratory Assessment Checklist for Blood Bank and Transfusion Services', states 'Specific policies regarding temperature control should be established and understood by all personnel. The major concern is the preservation of blood. If there is a power failure or refrigeration failure, arrangements must be made for urgent service and, if necessary, for alternative storage of blood'. The questions which relate to the facilities rather than to procedures used in the management of the facilities are shown in Figure 7.9.

3. EQUIPMENT

Medical refrigeration equipment for the transport and storage of blood and blood products must conform to the relevant Australian Standards.

Specific policies regarding temperature control should be established and understood by all personnel. The major concern is the preservation of blood. If there is a power failure or refrigeration failure, arrangements must be made for urgent service and for alternative storage of blood and documented.

3.1 Cold Storage

3.1.1   Is the blood arranged in the refrigerator(s) so that
there can be no confusion regarding:

(i) blood group   YES ☐ NO ☐ N/A ☐

(ii) unprocessed blood   YES ☐ NO ☐ N/A ☐

(iii) blood suitable for cross matching   YES ☐ NO ☐ N/A ☐

(iv) crossmatched blood *etc.*

3.1.2   Do authorised persons other than laboratory
staff have access to blood stocks   YES ☐ NO ☐ N/A ☐

3.1.3   Is there documentation to ensure the
security of the refrigerator(s)   YES ☐ NO ☐ N/A ☐

3.1.4   Are stock control procedures carried out daily
to ensure efficient use of the blood held   YES ☐ NO ☐ N/A ☐

from NPAAC Laboratory Assessment Checklist. Blood Banks and Transfusion Services 1995

Figure 7.9 NPAAC Blood Bank and Transfusion Services – Cold storage

HEALTH, SAFETY AND WELFARE
'Ideal Standard' clause 6.6 Health, safety and welfare
There are now a number of ISO and other internationally used standards, concerned with health and safety and the environment, with potential application to the medical laboratory (Figure 7.10).

The standards on management of occupational health, safety and the environment focus on management issues, most of which can be incorporated in a general quality management system. The contents of ISO/DIS 15190 'Medical laboratories – requirements for safety management' are shown in Figure 7.11 and indicate its direct application to safety management in the medical laboratory.

Title of the standard	Application	Abbreviation used in text
ISO/DIS 15190 Medical laboratories – requirements for safety management	For safety management in medical laboratories	ISO/DIS 15190
OHSAS 18001:1999 Occupational health and safety management systems – Specifications	For occupational health and safety management	OHSAS 18001:1999
OHSAS 18002:2000 Occupational health and safety management systems – Guidelines for the implementation of OHSAS 18001	Guidelines for occupational health and safety management	OHSAS 18002:2000
ISO 14001:1996 Environmental management systems – Specification with guidance for use	For environmental management	ISO 14001:1996

Figure 7.10 Standards – Occupational health, safety and environment

In addition there are a wide range of publications, many available free of charge, from the Health and Safety Executive (HSE) in the UK which provide sound practical advice. These publications are cited, where relevant, throughout this book and details provided in Appendix 2, Further reading.

The European Community (EC) since its beginning has been concerned with the area of workers' safety. In the EC the implementation of the articles of a Treaty is accomplished by a number of different legislative processes amongst which is the promulgation of Directives. A Directive is important as it 'shall be binding, as to the result to be achieved, upon each Member State to which it is addressed, but shall leave it to national authorities the choice of form and methods' of implementation (the principle of subsidiarity, see Chapter 2).

In the Single European Act of 1987 there are two articles which relate to Health and Safety. Article 100a requires harmonization of national legislation and seeks the removal of barriers to trade that can be caused by different national safety standards. Article 118a, requires the harmonization of existing Health and Safety laws throughout the EC stating in clause 1 that, 'Member States shall pay particular attention to encouraging improvements, especially in the working environment, as regards the health and safety of workers, and shall set as their objective the harmonization of conditions in this area, while maintaining the improvements made'.

4 Management requirements 4.1 Management responsibilities 4.2 Management of staff health	**12 Handwashing** **13 First aid and emergency** **practices**
5 Designing for safety 5.1 General design requirements 5.2 Physical considerations	**14 Good housekeeping practices** **15 Safe work practices with** **material of biological origin**
6 Staffing, procedures, documentation **inspection and records** 6.1 Laboratory safety officer 6.2 Procedures 6.3 Safety program audits 6.4 Safety manual 6.5 Records	**16 Aerosols** **17 Biological safety cabinets,** **chemical safety hoods and** **cupboards** **18 Chemical safety** **19 Radiation safety** 19.1 Radionuclides
7 Identification of hazards **8 Reporting of incidents, accidents** **and occupational illness** **9 Training**	19.2 UV and laser light sources 19.3 Microwave equipment **20 Fire precautions** 20.1 Construction
10 Personnel responsibilities 10.1 Food, drink and like substances 10.2 Cosmetics, hair, beards and jewellery	20.2 Secondary exits 20.3 Alarm systems 20.4 Fire risk reduction strategies
11 Clothing, personal protective **equipment (PPE)** 11.1 Laboratory protective clothing 11.2 Face and body protection 11.3 Gloves 11.4 Footwear 11.5 Respiratory protection	20.5 Storage of inflammable materials 20.6 Fire safety training programmes 20.7 Fire fighting equipment **21 Emergency evacuations** **22 Electrical equipment** **23 Transport of samples** **24 Waste disposal**

Adapted from ISO/DIS 15190 Medical laboratories - Requirements for safety management

Figure 7.11 The provisions of ISO/DIS 15190

In 1989, Directive 89/391/EEC introduced measures to encourage improvements in the safety and health of workers at work. The Directive had a general provision that the employer bears the duty to ensure the safety and health of workers in every aspect related to the workplace and the main principles are summarised in

Figure 7.12. Article (16) 1 of this 'framework Directive' required that, following its introduction, further individual Directives must be adopted and reference will be made to them at relevant places in the text.

- The employer must ensure that an assessment is made of the risks to health and safety at work.

- The employer must ensure that the workers of the undertaking receive information on, among other things, the safety and health risks, preventive measures, first aid, fire fighting and risk assessments.

- The employer must consult workers and/or their representatives on matters concerning their safety and health.

- The employer must ensure that each worker receives adequate and job-specific safety and health training.

- Each worker has an obligation to take care of his/her own safety and health and to make correct use of machinery, dangerous substances, personal protective clothing, etc.

based on William Hunter, Social Europe 3/93 'Europe for safety and health at work' 1989

Figure 7.12 Main principles of the Directive 89/391/EEC on health and safety

The requirements and inter-relationships of clause 6.6 'Health, safety and welfare' of the 'Ideal Standard' are shown in Figure 7.13.

The remainder of the chapter looks at the organization and management of health and safety. It is not, however, intended to be an authoritative guide to all aspects of the subject.

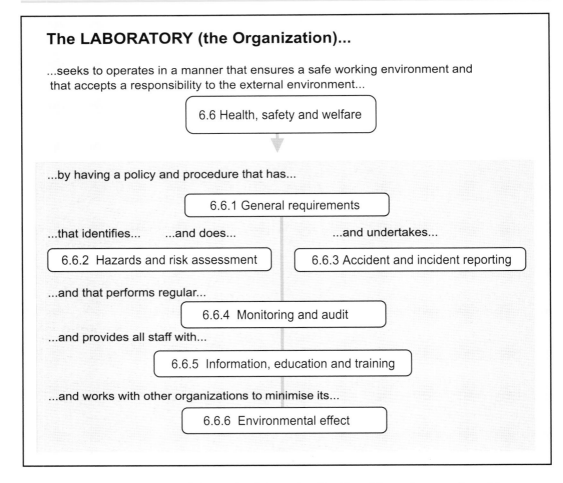

The LABORATORY (the Organization)...

...seeks to operates in a manner that ensures a safe working environment and that accepts a responsibility to the external environment...

6.6 Health, safety and welfare

...by having a policy and procedure that has...

6.6.1 General requirements

...that identifies...   ...and does...   ...and undertakes...

6.6.2 Hazards and risk assessment   6.6.3 Accident and incident reporting

...and that performs regular...

6.6.4 Monitoring and audit

...and provides all staff with...

6.6.5 Information, education and training

...and works with other organizations to minimise its...

6.6.6 Environmental effect

Figure 7.13 Clause 6.6 of the 'Ideal Standard' – Health, safety and welfare

GENERAL REQUIREMENTS
'Ideal Standard' clause 6.6.1 General requirements
The content of the procedure for the organization and management of health, safety and welfare in the laboratory of St Elsewhere's is shown in Figure 7.14. Certain issues will be developed in concert with the parent body or host organization, but the majority of the issues are specific to the laboratory.

HEALTH AND SAFETY POLICY STATEMENT
In many countries it is a legal requirement that every employer (except where less than five people are employed) must prepare and, as often as may be appropriate, revise a written statement of the general policy with respect to the health and safety at work of employees and of any other person entering the workplace, and the organization and arrangements for carrying out that policy. This statement

and any revisions must be brought to the attention of all employees. The policy statement of St Elsewhere's Hospital Trust is shown in Figure 7.15. This general policy statement forms the second item in the Health and Safety Handbook (Figure 7.17) and is contained in the procedure for the organization and management of health and safety (Figure 7.14). In addition to this statement the procedure requires the preparation of a Health and Safety Handbook which would be a major vehicle for communication to employees.

---

0 INTRODUCTION

    0.1 Purpose and scope

    0.2 Responsibility

    0.3 References

    0.4 Definitions

    0.5 Documentation

1 ORGANIZATION AND MANAGEMENT

    1.1 General

    1.2 Management/employer

    1.3 Workers representative(s)

    1.4 Workers/employees

    1.5 Health and safety officer

2 HEALTH AND SAFETY COMMITTEE

    2.1 Officers and membership

    2.2 Frequency of meetings

    2.3 Agenda

    2.4 Minutes

3 DOCUMENTATION

    3.1 Health and Safety Policy Statement

        [MF-GEN-H&SPol]

    3.2 Health and Safety Handbook

        [MF-GEN-H&SHbk]

    3.3 Forms and records

        [MF-GEN-H&SAud]

4 LABELLING OF HAZARDS

5 RISK ASSESSMENT

6 ACCIDENT AND INCIDENT REPORTING

7 MONITORING AND AUDIT

    [MF-GEN-H&SAud]

Figure 7.14 Contents of a procedure for the organization and management of health and safety [MP-GEN-H&SMan]

RESPONSIBILITIES

EMPLOYER/MANAGEMENT

The EC 'framework directive' (Figure 7.12), has a general provision that the employer has the overall responsibility for health and safety in the workplace and Article 6 which deals with general obligations for employers says '...the employer shall take measures necessary for the safety and health protection of workers, including the prevention of occupational risks and provision of information and training, as well as provision of the necessary organization and means'.

Although the overall organization and management of health and safety lies with the employer, the successful implementation and maintenance of any policy depends on co-operation of all the personnel in the laboratory. An understanding of the responsibilities of the different parties is extremely important, and includes, in addition to the employer, the employees' representative(s), the workers or employees, and the Health and Safety Officer. Each member of staff should have a clear reporting line with regard to health and safety matters. The parent body or host organization may also have a Fire Officer or advice from the local fire service, trained first aiders and an occupational health department.

The Health and Safety Policy of St Elsewhere's Hospital Trust

1. The Trust recognises that the safety of all its employees and other persons on its premises is of paramount importance and accepts its responsibility for providing a safe and healthy workplace.

2. The Trust will meet its responsibility, so far as is reasonably practical, paying particular attention to the provision and maintenance of:

   - safe place of work with safe access to and from it
   - a healthy working environment
   - plant, equipment and systems of work which are safe
   - safe arrangements for the use, handling, storage and transport of articles and substances
   - sufficient information, instruction, training and supervision to enable employees to avoid hazards and contribute positively to their own health and safety at work

3. The Trust undertakes the systematic identification of hazards, the recording of any significant risks arising from them, the establishment of arrangements to eliminate, reduce or control risks, and procedures for the review and revision of these arrangements.

4. The Trust will appoint safety officers competent to provide health and safety advice and assistance and deal with emergencies and situations of imminent danger to health and safety.

5. The Trust will co-operate fully in the appointment of safety representatives and will provide them, where necessary, with sufficient facilities and training to carry out this task.

6. The Trust will ensure the existence of a Health and Safety Committee.

7. A copy of this statement will be brought to the attention of all employees. It will be reviewed, or modified from time to time and may be supplemented in appropriate cases by further statements relating to the work of particular groups of employees.

Anne Braithwaite   22nd April 1999

The Chief Executive of St Elsewhere's Hospital Trust

Figure 7.15   The health and safety policy of St Elsewhere's Hospital Trust

WORKERS REPRESENTATIVE

Article 11 of the EC 'framework directive' on consultation (with) and participation (of) workers states that 'employers shall consult workers and/or their representatives and allow them to take part in discussions on all questions relating to safety and health at work' and requires employers among other things, to allow 'adequate time off work, without loss of pay, and provide them with the necessary means to enable such representatives to exercise their rights and functions deriving from the Directive'. Such representatives have a valuable role to play in any well run laboratory. They could be members of the Health and Safety Committee, or report to it.

WORKERS/EMPLOYEES

In most legislation on health and safety, not only does the employer/management have the overall responsibility, but also the workers themselves have responsibilities. Article 13 of the 'framework Directive' states, 'It shall be the responsibility of each worker to take care, as far as possible, of his* own safety and health and that of other persons affected by his acts or omissions at work in accordance with his training and instructions given by his employer'. To this end it requires workers to make correct use of work equipment and personal protective equipment, to have due regard to safety devices, to co-operate with the employer or worker representatives and to inform them of any work situation that they consider to represent a serious and immediate danger to health and safety.

LABORATORY SAFETY OFFICER

In Article 7, 'Protective and preventive services', it states that the 'employer shall designate one or more workers to carry out activities related to the protection and prevention of occupational risks for the undertaking and/or establishment'. Alternatively in the absence of competent personnel 'the employer shall enlist competent external services or persons'. Pathology laboratories should have a designated safety officer or officers. It is important that all staff understand the role of the safety officer and where it begins and ends (Figure 7.16). In particular it is important to understand that diminution or termination of risk is a management responsibility.

---

*The wording of the directive uses 'his' but it would read better as 'their' and 'the' as appropriate.

A laboratory safety officer should be appointed by management to...

- provide guidance to management and supervisors

- propose a safety programme and provide safety expertise

- propose, provide or obtain safety training

- serve ex-officio on the Health and Safety committee

- carry out risk assessments and recommend action as required

- stop activities that are unsafe and be authorized by management to do so

...but diminution or termination of risk is a management responsibility

---

Figure 7.16 The role of a laboratory safety officer

HEALTH AND SAFETY COMMITTEE
At St Elsewhere's the Health and Safety Committee is chaired by a member of the Pathology Management Board. The chairman could either be the Director of Pathology or a senior person to whom the responsibility is delegated. Its primary function is to ensure that procedures for the organization and management of health and safety are implemented. The Laboratory Safety Officer is an important member of the Health and Safety Committee but functions better by not having the dual role of chairman and officer. In addition to workers representatives, the committee has representatives from each department in pathology so that all issues are represented (including office staff). Although the committee has the important role to co-ordinate health and safety, every member of staff must understand their responsibilities as individuals that form part of their job descriptions (Figure 6.7).

DOCUMENTATION – THE LABORATORY HEALTH AND SAFETY MANUAL
The contents of the laboratory health and safety handbook (MP-GEN-H&SHbk) at St Elsewhere's Hospital are shown in Figure 7.17.

The detailed content will be determined by what else is available in the rest of the organization, local rules, guidelines, codes of practice, and regulations. The style of presentation and accessibility of the handbook is important if it is to be used for the education and training of staff and management. The Health and Safety Policy statement could either be that of the laboratory or of the parent body or host organization. All new employees are required to read the handbook as part of their induction training and are examined as to their understanding of its contents. In many countries the governmental organizations responsible for the inspection of health, safety and welfare in the workplace produce valuable informative literature regarding the handling of certain situations (see Appendix 2, Further reading).

1	**GENERAL INTRODUCTION**	**5**	**PERSONAL PROTECTIVE EQUIPMENT**
2	**THE HEALTH AND SAFETY POLICY**		5.1 Protective clothing
3	**MAINTENANCE OF HEALTH AND SAFETY IN THE LABORATORY**		5.2 Face and body protection
			5.3 Gloves
	3.1 Responsibilities		5.4 Footware
	3.2 Procedures and records		5.5 Respiratory protection
	3.3 Identification of hazards and risk assessment	**6**	**FIRST AID AND EMERGENCY PROVISION**
	3.4 Warning signs and labels	**7**	**GOOD HOUSEKEEPING**
	3.5 Health and safety audits	**8**	**SAFE WORKING PRACTICES**
	3.6 Reporting of incidents, accidents and occupational illness		8.1 Biological materials
			8.2 Chemicals
	3.7 Training		8.3 Carcinogens
4	**PERSONAL HYGIENE AND RESPONSIBILITIES**		8.4 Radionuclides and other radiation sources
	4.1 Smoking, food and drink and substance use		8.5 Compressed gases
			8.6 Electrical equipment
	4.2 Cosmetics, hair, beards and jewellery		8.7 Waste management
		9	**FIRE PRECAUTIONS**
	4.3 Handwashing	**10**	**EMERGENCY EVACUATIONS**

Figure 7.17 Contents of the Health and Safety handbook at St Elsewhere's laboratory (MP-GEN-H&SHbk)

The responsibility for its production and updating is clearly defined in the procedure for health and safety management (MP-GEN-H&SMan) (Figure 7.14) and it is subject to the document control procedures described in Chapter 5.

In the UK the Health Service Advisory Committee of the UK Health and Safety Commission has produced a series of model rules for staff and visitors which could be included in the Health and Safety handbook as appendices, or preferably, free standing posters. They include model rules for clinical, scientific, technical and medical laboratory staff, phlebotomists and venepuncturists, laboratory office staff, laboratory reception staff, laboratory porters and messengers, cleaning staff in the laboratory (domestic and ancillary), maintenance staff and equipment service engineers in clinical laboratories, and for visitors to laboratories. As an example the model rules for laboratory office staff are shown in Figure 7.18. It is a controlled document [MF-GEN-H&SOffR]

Rules for laboratory office staff

Most of the work in the laboratory is concerned with the handling of specimens that may be infectious. Office staff are not required to come into direct contact with these materials, but may accidently do so when handling bags and packages containing specimens. Such workers, in addition to following the general precautions outlined above, should also take the following safety measures.

(a) If you work in an office that has direct access into the laboratory, wear a coat or gown, like the other laboratory staff.

(b) Wash your hands after you have been into the laboratory and may have come into contact with laboratory items or materials that could be infectious.

(c) Never lick stamps or labels. Use a roller pad, damp sponge or self-adhesive labels.

(d) If you are required to package specimens, only do so if the containers are in a sealed transport bag. If there is any sign of breakage or leakage do not touch the bag. Report it to your supervisor immediately.

'Safe working and the prevention of infection in clinical laboratories - model rules for staff and visitors'
Health Service Advisory Committee of the Health and Safety Commission (UK) 1991

Figure 7.18 Model rules for laboratory office staff

The NCCLS Document, M29-A2 'Protection of Laboratory Workers from Occupationally Acquired Infections', published in 2001, represents a valuable resource on this topic. It aims to promote 'the essence of good laboratory practice to protect workers from infectious diseases in the work place'. One of the key defences against infection is the concept of 'Standard Precautions' (formerly known as universal precautions), which requires that 'all patients and all laboratory specimens should be handled as if they are capable of transmitting disease'. M29-A2 delineates the components: a) thorough handwashing whether or not gloves are worn, b) the wearing of gloves and gowns, c) the wearing of 'a mask, eye protection or a face shield to protect the mucous membranes of the eyes, nose and mouth during procedures that are likely to generate splashes or sprays of blood or other potentially infectious diseases', d) the proper handling of potentially infected equipment or devices, e) to 'ensure that the laboratory has adequate procedures for the routine care, cleaning and disinfection of environment surfaces and frequently touched items' and f) proper procedures for handling 'sharps'. The section on 'Standard Precautions' concludes by arguing that these precautions, 'eliminate the need for using specific biohazard warnings on specimens obtained from patients infected with HBV, HIV and other pathogens, including antibiotic resistant organisms'.

DOCUMENTATION – FORMS AND CHECKLISTS
The forms and checklists used in risk assessment, monitoring and audit and incident reporting are described in the sections below. It is these completed forms and checklists, together with the minutes of the Health and Safety Committee, that represent the records which can be referred to at a quality or accreditation inspection to establish compliance with procedures.

HAZARDS AND RISK ASSESSMENT
'Ideal Standard' clause 6.6.2 Hazards and risk assessment
The process of risk assessment requires the identification of hazards. They can arise from the activities taking place in the laboratory or from other factors such as the layout of the laboratory. A hazard can be defined as 'something with the potential to do harm', and can include for example, chemical substances, biological agents, equipment or methods of working. The term risk is 'the likelihood that some harm can come from the particular hazard', and the extent of risk means the number of people who might be exposed to the hazard and the consequences for them.

Article 6 of the 'framework Directive' includes among the general obligations on employers the requirement that they shall 'evaluate the risks to the safety and health of the workers, inter alia in the choice of work equipment, the chemical substances or preparation used, and the fitting out of workplaces'. The requirement to evaluate risks to workers is a continuing theme in subsequent directives. 'Use of work equipment' (Directive 89/655/EEC of 30 November 1989), 'Use of personal protective equipment' (Directive 89/656/EEC of 30 November 1989), 'Use of display screen equipment' (Directive 90/270/EEC of 29 May 1990) and the 'Manual handling of loads' (Directive 90/269/EEC of 29 May 1990), all of which have application in the pathology laboratory.

In most countries there are also regulations concerning the use of chemical and biological agents, carcinogens (including a prohibition list) and radioisotopes (in vitro and in vivo). In all these areas the requirement is an evaluation of the risks to workers and the sharing of the results with the staff involved. The hazards to be evaluated range from a filing cabinet being unstable when the drawers are open, to the handling of samples which might contain HIV.

In the EC, and in other legislatures, the evaluation of risk is a legal requirement. If an employer has difficulty in understanding how to undertake risk evaluations, the local Health and Safety Inspectorate can provide information on relevant publications. The Health and Safety Executive (UK) has prepared a leaflet to guide the process entitled 'Five steps to risk assessment'. It is important for whoever is undertaking the risk assessment, whether it is the employer himself or a person designated to do it on his behalf, such as a Health and Safety Officer or an outside expert, to follow the steps recommended. As this concept of risk assessment is becoming increasingly important, particularly with regard to acceptance for insurance, further advice regarding each step is summarised in Figure 7.19.

In the next chapter the responsibilities of manufacturers in relation to the IVD Directive are discussed and one result of that Directive is the publication of prEN 13641:2001, 'Elimination or reduction of risk of infection related to in vitro diagnostic reagents', which requires manufacturers to seek the elimination or reduction of risk of infection related to in vitro diagnostic reagents. More advice on risk assessment in relation to pre-examination, examination and post-examination processes is given in Chapters 9 & 10.

ACCIDENT AND INCIDENT REPORTING
'Ideal Standard' clause 6.6.3 Accident and incident reporting
Even when effective risk assessment has been completed in a laboratory and the appropriate steps have been taken to minimise the risk associated with the hazards identified, inevitably there will still be incidents such as 'needle stick' injuries. It is an important part of health and safety procedure that these incidents are recorded and an investigation carried out to determine whether the risk can be further reduced. This may require changes in particular procedures or improvements in the training given to staff.

All incidents should be recorded and evaluated as part of the health and safety procedure, but additionally in many countries there is a legal requirement to report certain injuries, diseases and dangerous occurrences to the appropriate enforcing authority for record and, if appropriate, investigation. Which incidents constitute reportable events will vary between countries, but Figure 7.20 shows a typical categorisation in connection with 'The Reporting of Injuries, Diseases and Dangerous Occurences Regulations' (RIDDOR) 1995, in the UK, with examples which are appropriate to a laboratory situation.

Step 1 Look for the hazards

- Walk around your laboratory and look afresh at what could reasonably be expected to cause harm.
- Ignore the trivial and concentrate on significant hazards which could result in serious harm or affect several people.
- Ask your employees or their representatives what they think. They may have noticed things which are not immediately obvious.
- Manufacturer's instructions or datasheets can also help you spot hazards and put risks in their true perspective. So can accident and ill-health records.

Step 2 Decide who might be harmed and how

- As well as people who work in the laboratory all the time, think about people who work there occasionally, e.g. cleaners, visitors, contractors, maintenance personnel, etc.
- Include members of the public if there is a chance they could be hurt by your activities.

Step 3 Evaluate the risks arising from the hazards and decide whether existing precautions are adequate or more should be done

- Even after all precautions have been taken, some risk usually remains. What you have to decide for each significant hazard is whether this remaining risk is high, medium or low.
- First, ask yourself whether you have done all the things that the law or a code of good practice says you have got to do e.g. guidance regarding the wearing of protective clothing whilst using disinfectants in mortuaries.
- Then ask yourself whether generally accepted standards are in place e.g. provision of protective clothing and training in its use.
- But don't stop there - think about yourself as an employer, because the law also says that you must do what is reasonably practicable to keep your laboratory safe.
- Your real aim is to make all risks small by adding to your precautions if necessary.

Step 4 Record your findings

- You must record the significant findings of your assessment by (1) writing down the more significant hazards and (2) recording your most important conclusions e.g. use of disinfectants in the mortuary: protective clothing provided and training given.
- You must also inform your employees about your findings.
- Assessments need to be suitable and sufficient, not perfect. The real points are: are the precautions reasonable, and is there something to show that a proper chack was made?
- Keep the written document for future reference or use; it can help you if an inspector questions your precautions, or if you become involved in any action for civil liability. It can also remind you to keep an eye on particular matters. And it helps to show that you have done what the law requires.
- To make things simpler, you can refer to other documents, such as manuals, the arrangements in your health and safety policy statement, manufacturer's instructions, and your health and safety procedures.

Step 5 Review your assessment from time to time and revise it if necessary

- Sooner or later you will bring in new apparatus, substances and procedures which could lead to new hazards. You should add to the assessment to take account of the new hazard.
- It is good practice to review your assessment from time to time.
- Don't amend your assessment for every trivial change, or still more, for each new activity, but if a new activity introduces significant new hazards of its own, you must consider them in their own right and do whatever you need to keep risks down.

based on 5 steps to Risk Assessment. Health and Safety Executive 1994

Figure 7.19 Five steps to risk assessment

Death or major injury

An accident connected with work and where your employee, or a self-employed person working on your premises, is killed or suffers a major injury (including as a result of physical violence); or a member of the public is killed or taken to hospital e.g.

- unconsciousness caused by asphyxia or exposure to a harmful substance or biological agent

- acute illness requiring medical treatment, or loss of consciousness arising from absorption of any substance by inhalation, ingestion or through the skin

- acute illness requiring medical treatment where there is reason to believe that this resulted from exposure to a biological agent or its toxins or infected material.

Over-three day injury

An accident connected with work (including an act of physical violence) and your employee, or a self-employed person working on your premises, suffers an over-three day injury. An over-three day injury is one which is not major but results in the injured person being away from work or unable to do their normal work for more than three days (including non-work days).

Disease

If a doctor notifies you that your employee suffers from a reportable work-related disease e.g.

- certain poisonings

- some skin conditions such as occupational dermatitis, skin cancer, chrome ulcer, oil folliculitis/acne

- infections such as: leptospirosis, hepatitis, tuberculosis, anthrax, legionellosis and tetanus.

Dangerous occurence

If something happens which does not result in a reportable injury, but clearly could have done, then it may be a dangerous occurence which must be reported e.g.

- accidental release of a biological agent likely to cause severe human illness

- accidental release of any substance which can damage health.

based on Reporting of Injuries, Disease and Dangerous Occurences Regulations 1995
Health and Safety Executive UK

Figure 7.20   Categories of reportable incidents

Reporting in the UK can be via www.riddor.gov.uk. or using Microsoft Word templates that can be downloaded from the website. Advice is also given on in-house records, 'you must keep a record of any reportable injury, disease or dangerous occurrence. This must include the date and method of reporting; the date, time and place of the event, personal details of those involved and a brief description of the nature of the event or disease. You can keep the record in any form you wish'.

One of the major problems with all aspects of health and safety is how to maintain interest in a topic which staff may regard as an extra imposition on an already busy day. How often do laboratory staff attend fire lectures with enthusiasm! Making the process as simple and streamlined as possible goes a long way to ensuring staff participation.

MONITORING AND AUDIT
'Ideal Standard' clause 6.6.4 Monitoring and audit
The process of monitoring and audit has similarities with risk assessment. However, monitoring and audit has more to do with compliance with the advised precautionary measures, for example laboratory staff wearing protective clothing when appropriate, as distinct from the provision of protective clothing as a response to a risk assessment. At St Elsewhere's, two comprehensive health and safety audits (plus four on special topics) are carried out annually and the reports presented to workers/representatives and the Pathology Management Board. These reports also form part of the annual management review (Chapter 11). The minutes of the Board should record acceptance of the audits and their response to any recommendations. In order that nothing of importance is missed audits are best carried out against a check list which can also serve to provide a record of the audit. A useful basis for a check list can be the laboratory safety sections of inspection check lists of accreditation schemes. Such material, is available from the College of American Pathology website (www.cap.org) in Word, .html or .pdf format. In the CAP-LAP Inspection Checklist – Laboratory General, Section I (Sept 2002), questions are included on the general safety programme for the whole laboratory. It is divided into two sections; the first involves questions concerning 'manuals and records', and the second the 'physical inspection of the laboratory'.

A major area for monitoring and audit should be 'good housekeeping', and at St Elsewhere's a technique for undertaking such an audit is used in a two hour training programme for ten people. Participants are invited to prepare, without discussion, a list of five questions that they feel should be on a checklist for a 'Good Housekeeping Audit' (15 minutes). After discussion the group create a checklist of the ten most important items (30 minutes), and then go in pairs, one senior and one junior person, to undertake the audit (30 minutes) in an area specified by the course organizer. Finally they return to discuss the results and decide on agreed action and timescales (45 minutes). Figure 7.21 illustrates this activity.

'GOOD HOUSEKEEPING' AUDIT TRAINING FORM			
RECORD FILENAME		*MF-GEN-H&SAudTra*	
1 Auditers	*George O'Kelly/Tim Hewitt*	**2 Position**	*Trainee Biochemist/Computer Manager*
3 Location of audit	*Biochemistry-Routine laboratory*	**4 Date of course**	*10th May 2002*

5 Items for audit		
Enter below the top ten items for audit	**Enter observations**	**Enter action to be taken and time scale where possible**
1. *Examine whether the floor is cluttered with unnecessary items*	*Under the on-call bench there were a number of empty cardboard boxes*	*Dispose of immediately*
2. *Check shelves for items no longer in use*	*Shelf above the on-call bench had used reagent containers in cardboard box and out of date internal quality control materials*	*Dispose of boxes immediately and ask the routine section supervisor to check which batch of internal quality control material is currently being used*
3. *Is the floor covering in good condition without cracks?*	*The floor covering has been recently replaced but near the on-call bench it was splattered with blood*	*Ensure that this area is cleaned properly*
4. *Are there plug borders in use or multi-adapters on electric points?*	*No*	*N/a*
5. *Are the notice boards kept well organized and up to date?*	*Excellent well organised notice boards for staff information*	*N/a*
6. *Are there laboratory instructions stuck on the walls or on equipment - and if so are they controlled documents?*	*The instructions for use of the blood gas analyser [MI-BIO-BlGas341] were stuck on the wall with Blu® tack and the review date was Jan 3rd 2002*	*Check whether the review date for [MI-BIO-BlGas341] had been missed and take appropriate action immediately*
7. *Are supplies of protective gloves readily available?*	*Yes and well labelled*	*N/a*
8. *Is the fire equipment in place and has it been inspected within the last year?*	*All fire equipment in place and last checked on February 4th 2002*	*N/a*
9. *Are the working surfaces clear of unnecessary paperwork?*	*The area around the on-call bench was covered with used paper and unfiled maintenance/internal control sheets*	*All completed record sheets should be properly filed.*
10. *Are the clinical waste containers clearly marked?*	*Yes*	*N/a*

6 General recommendation
This brief audit reveals a number of problems in the area of the on-call bench, all of which can be taken care of immediately . These observations indicate a lack of proper management responsibility and it was discovered that the designated individual has been away on extended sick leave. Recommend that there be a designated deputy and internal monitoring by the supervisor of the routine laboratory to prevent a re-occurrence of these problems.

Figure 7.21 An exercise in 'good housekeeping' audit

Monitoring should be seen as an ongoing formal, or informal process, of checking compliance to understood and promulgated standards. It might, for example, involve gentle but firm reminders to heads of departments that they too should wear protective clothing in the 'dirty' areas of the laboratory! In addition to internal monitoring and audit, inspectors from the appropriate government agency will make visits from time to time and present a report in which any noncompliances to regulations or codes of practice are listed. The employer/management will have to respond in a given period and satisfy the inspectorate that remedial action has been taken. Occasionally a noncompliance might be serious enough to require immediate suspension of a particular activity.

INFORMATION, EDUCATION AND TRAINING
'Ideal Standard' clause 6.6.5 Information, education and training
An important part of creating a good 'health and safety culture' is the education and training provided. Any courses such as the 'good housekeeping' audit training, previously described, should be recorded in personnel training records (see Figure 6.17). The important factor in education and training is to make it relevant to the individual's particular situation. If a member of staff has to move heavy gas cylinders then for that individual a course in manual handling would be relevant and meaningful. A useful approach is to design material that encourages members of staff to evaluate their own work situation and Government Agencies responsible for Health and Safety often have useful material available. A good example is a pamphlet, 'Working with VDUs', produced by the Health and Safety Executive (UK) which provides information concerning the UK regulations which were developed in response to EC Directive, 90/270/EEC of 29 May 1990, on 'Use of display screen equipment'. In addition to answering questions about health matters, it outlines the regulations and what employers have to do to comply, and finishes with a section entitled 'What can I do to help myself?' (Figure 7.22).

ENVIRONMENTAL EFFECT
'Ideal Standard' clause 6.6.6 Environment effect
In a previous section requirements for the environment within the workplace were discussed, but in this section a broader definition is required. This broader concept has been defined as, 'the surroundings and conditions in which an organization operates, including living systems (human and other) therein. As the environmental effects of the organization may reach all parts of the world, the environment in this context extends from the workplace to the global system'. The discovery of specific radioactive isotopes in sheep on the Welsh hills which relate to the emissions caused by the Chernobyl disaster are a graphic reminder of the environment as a global system. The ISO standard, ISO 14001:1996, 'Environmental management systems – Specification with guidance for use on environmental management', is one of a series of publications on all aspects of environmental management.

WHAT CAN I DO TO HELP MYSELF?

Make full use of the equipment provided and adjust it to get the best from it and avoid potential health problems. If the Regulations apply to you, your employer should cover these things in training. If the Regulations don't apply to you, it is still worth setting up your workstation properly, to be as comfortable as possible.

Here are some practical tips:

Getting comfortable...

- Adjust your chair and VDU to find the most comfortable position for your work. As a broad guide, your forearms should be approximately horizontal and your eyes at the same height as the top of the VDU.
- Make sure you have enough workspace to take whatever documents or other equipment you have.
- Try different arrangements of keyboard, mouse and documents to find the best arrangement for you. A document holder may help you avoid awkward neck and eye movements.
- Arrange your desk and VDU to avoid glare, or bright reflections on the screen. This will be easiest if neither you or the screen are directly facing windows or bright lights. Adjust curtains or blinds to prevent unwanted light.
- Make sure there is enough space underneath your desk to move your legs freely. Move any obstacles such as boxes or equipment.
- Avoid excess pressure on the backs of your legs or knees. A footrest, particularly for smaller users, may be helpful.

Keying in...

- Adjust your keyboard to get a good keying in position. A space in front of the keyboard is sometimes helpful for resting the hands and wrists when not keying.
- Try to keep your wrists straight when keying, Keep a soft touch on the keys and don't overstretch your fingers. Good keyboard technique is important.

Using the mouse...

- Position the mouse within easy reach, so that it can be used with the wrist straight. Sit upright and close to the desk, so you don't have to work with your mouse arm outstretched. Move the keyboard out of the way if it is not being used.
- Support your forearm on the desk and don't grip the mouse too tightly.
- Rest your fingers lightly on the buttons and do not press them hard.

Reading the screen...

- Adjust the brightness and contrast controls on the screen to suit the lighting conditions in the room.
- Make sure the screen surface is clean.
- In setting up the software, choose options giving text that is large enough to read easily on the screen, when you are working in a normal, comfortable position. Select colours that are easy on the eye (avoid red text on a blue background or vice versa).
- Individual characters on the screen should be sharply focused and should not flicker or move. If they do, the VDU may need servicing.

Postures and breaks...

- Don't sit in the same position for long periods. Make sure you change your position as often as practicable. Some movement is desirable, but avoid repeated stretching to reach things you need (if this happens a lot rearrange your workstation).
- Most jobs provide opportunities to take a break from the screen e.g. to do some filing or copying. Make use of them. If there are no such natural breaks in your job, your employer should plan for you to have rest breaks. Frequent short breaks are better than a few long ones.

based on 'Working with VDUs' Health and Safety Executive UK 1998

Figure 7.22   Use of display screen equipment – 'What can I do to help myself?'

Many aspects of the management environmental effects are illustrated in Figure 7.23. One aspect, pertinent to the pathology laboratory is the requirement to have procedures for waste management, and this is included in the contents of the Laboratory Health and Safety Handbook (Figure 7.17). It is important that either the pathology laboratory and/or its parent body should develop procedures to manage resources efficiently and to minimise detrimental effects they may have on the external environment.

1. Assessment, control and reduction of the impact of the activity concerned on the various sections of the environment.

2. Energy management, savings and choice.

3. Raw materials management, savings, choice and transportation; water management and savings.

4. Waste avoidance, recycling, reuse, transportation and disposal.

5. Evaluation, control and reduction of noise within and outside the site.

6. Selection of new production processes and changes to production processes.

7. Product planning (design, packaging, transportation, use and disposal).

8. Environmental performance and practices of contractors, sub-contractors and suppliers.

9. Prevention and limitation of environmental accidents.

10. Contingency procedures in cases of environmental accidents.

11. Staff information and training on environmental issues.

12. External information on environmental issues.

modified from Annex 1 Council Regulations (EEC) No 1836/93 (1993)

Figure 7.23 Approaches to the management of environmental effects

In many countries there will be legislation regarding such matters as the disposal of hazardous waste, and the control of emissions into the atmosphere. In the UK, NHS Estates, an Executive Agency of the Department of Health, in conjunction with other bodies, has published a compendium of good practice on Healthcare Waste Minimisation that can be a useful starting point for a laboratory wishing to explore this area.

Chapter 8

Equipment and diagnostic systems (IVDs), and data and information systems

INTRODUCTION

'Ideal Standard' clause 6.4 Equipment and diagnostic systems (IVDs)/ 6.5 Data and information systems

This chapter looks at the procurement and provision of In Vitro medical diagnostic Devices (IVDs) and their management. Before proceeding with the general discussion it is important to define what is meant by the relatively new term, IVD.

In ISO 15189:2002, a note to the clause 5.3 *'Laboratory equipment'*, defines laboratory equipment as 'instruments, reference materials, consumables, reagents and analytical systems', in fact all items required for pre-examination, examination and, where appropriate, post-examination procedures. Within the EC Directive 98/79/EEC on *'in vitro* diagnostic medical devices' (IVDs), an IVD is defined as shown in Figure 8.1. For brevity this Directive is referred to as the IVD Directive in the rest of the chapter.

The term **'*in vitro* diagnostic medical device'** means...

'any medical device which is a reagent, reagent product, calibrator, control material, kit, instrument, apparatus, equipment, or system, whether used alone or in combination, intended by the manufacturer to be used *in vitro* for the examination of specimens, including blood and tissue donations, derived from the human body, solely or principally for the purpose of providing information:

- concerning a physiological or pathological state

- concerning a congenital abnormality

- to determine the safety and compatibility with potential recipients

- to monitor therapeutic measures'

based on EC Directive 98/79 EEC '*In vitro* diagnostic medical devices'

Figure 8.1 Definition of an 'in vitro diagnostic medical device'

It will become apparent later in the chapter why the IVD Directive will not only affect the EC countries, but also any manufacturer or supplier of medical laboratories to the EC. IVDs are a subset of Medical Devices and are distinguished from other Medical Devices, such as an ECG instrument, by not coming in direct contact with the patient. In some areas there is some uncertainty as to what should and should not be included in this definition. However as a general rule, and in the context of this book, anything used in a laboratory which contributes to the performance of an examination or analysis used in diagnosis, or that influences treatment, can be regarded as an IVD. In this context any computer system (hardware and software) used as a laboratory information system or in an analytical system would be regarded as an IVD, and in this chapter, all that is said concerning IVDs has potential application to computers in the laboratory.

In terms of ISO 9001:2000, ISO 17025:1999 and ISO 15189:2002, this chapter embraces two major issues, those relating to purchasing and supplies, (ISO 9001:2000, clause 7.4 *'Purchasing'*; ISO 17025:1999, clause 4.6 *'Purchasing supplies and services'*; and ISO 15189:2002, clause 4.6 *'External services and supplies'*) and those relating to requirements for IVDs, (ISO 9001:2000, clause 6.3 *'Infrastructure'*; ISO 17025:1999, clause 5.5 *'Equipment'*; and ISO 15189:2002, clause 5.3 *'Laboratory equipment'*). In a discussion of data and information management later in the chapter, ISO 15189:2002, Annex B (informative) *'Laboratory Information Systems'* (LIS), relates to specific issues for the management of data and information.

In summary, the requirement is that there must be the equipment (IVDs) required for the correct performance of the tests (examinations), which must be validated as fit for purpose, and be operated by authorized personnel using up to date instructions. Each item of equipment must be uniquely identified and records of the equipment and its calibration and maintenance kept. The procedures for the procurement and management of these IVDs must be defined and controlled. It is also a requirement that, 'where the laboratory needs to use equipment outside its permanent control, that it shall ensure that the requirements of this International Standard are met'. In this chapter this phrase is interpreted to mean a laboratory's involvement in 'Point of Care Testing' (POCT).

In the 'Ideal Standard' the two aspects are combined and Figure 8.2 shows the interconnectivity between the clauses and sub-clauses relating to equipment and diagnostic systems and data and information systems. Planned procurement and management of IVDs provides evidence of their fitness to meet the needs and requirements of users. The proper recording and security of data and information, in relation to all laboratory processes, allows audit trails to be established that provide evidence that these needs have been met in a timely and effective manner.

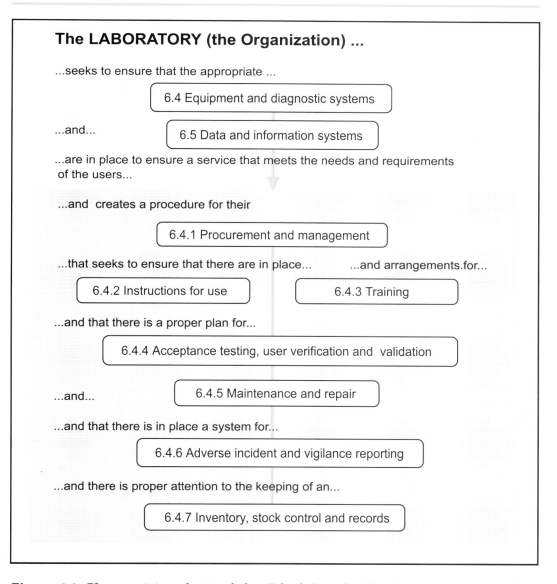

The LABORATORY (the Organization) ...

...seeks to ensure that the appropriate ...

> 6.4 Equipment and diagnostic systems

...and...

> 6.5 Data and information systems

...are in place to ensure a service that meets the needs and requirements of the users...

...and creates a procedure for their

> 6.4.1 Procurement and management

...that seeks to ensure that there are in place...   ...and arrangements.for...

> 6.4.2 Instructions for use   6.4.3 Training

...and that there is a proper plan for...

> 6.4.4 Acceptance testing, user verification and validation

...and...

> 6.4.5 Maintenance and repair

...and that there is in place a system for...

> 6.4.6 Adverse incident and vigilance reporting

...and there is proper attention to the keeping of an...

> 6.4.7 Inventory, stock control and records

Figure 8.2 Clauses 6.4 and 6.5 of the 'Ideal Standard' – Equipment and diagnostic systems (IVDs) and Data and information systems.

In the UK, the Medical Devices Agency (MDA), which is an Executive Agency of the Department of Health, is charged with safeguarding public health 'by working with users, manufacturers and lawmakers to ensure the medical devices meet appropriate standards of safety, quality and performance and that they comply with relevant Directives of the European Community (EC)'. In pursuance of this aim it has recently produced a Device Bulletin entitled, 'Management of *In*

Vitro Diagnostic Medical Devices' (referred to in the rest of this chapter as the MDA-DB-IVDs). This important document builds upon an earlier generic bulletin for Medical Devices, is freely available, and provides the structure of this chapter and of section 6.4 of the 'Ideal Standard'.

The IVD Directive is of particular importance, not only for the effect of its requirements on countries within the Community, but also because any manufacturer (or distributor/supplier) based outside the Community trading in the European Economic Area (the 15 EC member states plus Iceland, Norway and Liechtenstein) must comply with the regulations and CE (Conformité Européenne) marking of their devices. After 7 June 2003, manufacturers may not place on the market any IVD that does not have CE marking. CE marking indicates that the product to which it is affixed, conforms to all essential requirements and other applicable provisions that have been imposed upon it by European Directives and that the product has been subject to the appropriate conformity assessment procedure(s). The essential requirements refer, among other things to safety, public health and consumer protection.

The requirements of the IVD Directive on the manufacturer creates the opportunity for a partnership between the manufacturer and the purchasing laboratory. The manufacturer who fulfils the requirements of the IVD Directive and the medical laboratory seeking recognition of its performance through accreditation (as yet voluntary in many countries), are in a coalition that has the common aim of a quality service for the end user. Some key requirements for the manufacturer are shown in Figure 8.3.

The nature of the conformity assessment route will depend upon the nature of the IVD (see MDA-DB-IVDs for further information).

The **IVD Directive** introduces certain requirements (indicated by CE marking) on the manufacturer...

- The devices must be designed and manufactured in such a way that, when used under the conditions and for the purpose intended, they will not compromise, directly or indirectly, the clinical condition or the safety of the patients, the safety or health of users...

- The solutions adopted by the manufacturer for the design and construction of the devices must conform to safety principles, taking account of the generally acknowledged state of the art.

- ... they must achieve the performance, in particular, where appropriate, in terms of analytical sensitivity, diagnostic sensitivity, analytical specificity, diagnostic specificity, accuracy, repeatability, reproducibility, including control of known interferences, and limits of detection, stated by the manufacturer. 'The traceability of values assigned to calibrators and/or control materials must be assured through available reference measurement procedures and/or available reference materials of a higher order'.

- ...the manufacturer must have the data to demonstrate how the performance claims in terms of the above criteria have been established.

The **CE marking** process does not, however, demand clinical utility, that is for the purchaser (the medical laboratory).

based upon EC Directive 98/79 EEC on '*In vitro* diagnostic medical devices'

Figure 8.3 IVD Directive – some key requirements for the manufacturer

PROCUREMENT AND MANAGEMENT
'Ideal Standard' clause 6.4.1 Procurement and management
Pathology laboratories have a great diversity of IVDs, ranging from test tubes to large multichannel analyzers and sophisticated staining machines. Whether appropriate equipment is provided will be judged in relation to the type, work-load and purpose of the work undertaken by the laboratory. Simply stated, a blood glucose meter would not be appropriate for a large laboratory, but might be appropriate for 'point-of-care testing' on a ward.

For convenience in this book a distinction is made between 'equipment IVDs', items of equipment and major systems purchases, and smaller items termed 'consumable IVDs' such as reagents, quality control and calibration material, pipette tips etc. Sometimes the term 'IVD reagents' is used in standards, this is a subset of the term 'consumable IVDs'. A hard and fast separation is not possible because consumable and reagent items can also be an inherent part of an equipment purchase. The initial procurement process has to be the same regardless of the type of IVD, but the management of 'equipment IVDs' is evidenced more through an equipment inventory and maintenance and repair records whereas 'consumable IVDs' are managed through purchase, stock control and resulting records.

The purpose of IVD procurement and management is to ensure that they fulfil the requirements given in Figure 8.4. This is not the place to give a detailed account of IVD management, but in the discussion the importance of record keeping is emphasised. These records not only provide evidence that the procedure of procurement and management of IVDs is being followed, but also assist in the reconstruction of the audit trail associated with a particular examination. It is important to know from such records that a particular analyzer was in use at the time an examination was performed, that it had been serviced and calibrated and that the reagents, calibrators and internal quality control material used were in date and validated for use. The former lies in the remit of equipment inventories and the second in the area of stock control records.

Equipment procurement and management ensures that...

   a) it is suitable for its intended purpose

   b) its operation is understood by its users

   c) it is in a safe and proper operating condition

   d) it meets safety and quality standards and requirements

   e) it is stored or operated in appropriate and controlled conditions

   f) it satisfies a) to d) above in a cost effective manner

based on Health Equipment Information No.98 (1991) Management of Medical Equipment and Devices

---

Figure 8.4 Purpose of equipment procurement and management

In a recent external audit of St Elsewhere's Hospital, record keeping in relation to the procurement and management of larger items of laboratory equipment (equipment IVDs) was criticised and a new process is being trialed at the present time. The content of the new procedure is shown in Figure 8.5 and is being used in the purchase of new equipment, new computer systems and new sourcing of pre-poured plates in Microbiology. It covers a range of activities, some of which are dealt with by the laboratory and some, such as negotiation and purchase, that are done in accordance with the standing orders of the hospital.

---

0 INTRODUCTION
  0.1 Purpose and scope
  0.2 Responsibility
  0.3 References
  0.4 Definitions
  0.5 Documentation

1 PROCUREMENT OF EQUIPMENT IVDs
  1.1 Initiation of request [MF-GEN-IVDPrc]
  1.2 Assessment of need
  1.3 Market survey
  1.4 Collection of data
  1.5 Comparison of costs and features
  1.6 Negotiations and purchase
  1.7 Acceptance procedures [MF-GEN-IVDAcct]

2 MAINTENANCE AND REPAIR OF IVDs
  2.1 Maintenance contracts
  2.2 Decontamination and permit to work [MF-GEN-IVDServ]
  2.3 In house maintenance
  2.4 Records of maintenance and repair
  2.5 IVD equipment inventory
  2.6 Disposal

3 PURCHASE AND STOCK CONTROL OF CONSUMABLE IVDs

4 VALIDATION OF IVDs

5 DOCUMENTATION (INCLUDING INSTRUCTIONS FOR USE)

6 TRAINING
  6.1 Manufacturer/supplier training
  6.2 In house training including updates
  6.3 Records [MF-XXX-TrnRec]

7 ADVERSE INCIDENT REPORTING AND NOTIFICATION
  7.1 Internal reporting [MF-GEN-IVDRep]
  7.2 External reporting [MF-GEN-AdvIncd]

Figure 8.5 Contents of a procedure for the procurement and management of IVDs [MP-GEN-IVDPrc]

Procurement may involve the purchase of a new piece of equipment for new service, or the replacement of existing equipment with an identical piece of equipment or a later model. The brief description that follows is based upon the MDA Device Bulletin for 'Medical Device and Equipment Management for Hospital and Community-based organizations' and MDA-DB-IVDs. The process starts in consultation with the user, to establish the need for a new item or to reevaluate an existing service. For purposes of the present discussion the assumption is made that there is a request for a new test for the identification of myocardial infarction within 4 hours of the onset of chest pain that involves measuring levels of Myocard Z in plasma. It is agreed that the service should be available 24 hours per day and that results be returned within 20 minutes from the time the sample is taken. This immediately triggers numerous questions, where should the test be performed (in the laboratory or as a point-of-care test), by whom, (nurses and doctors or laboratory staff), etc all of which must be considered in the *'assessment of need'* that is then recorded. The next step is to carry out a *'market survey'* to identify the manufacturers/suppliers who can potentially provide systems that are fit for the purpose. Then for each manufacturer/supplier there needs to be *'collection of data'*. This data includes financial data and technical specifications, evaluation reports, user experience and information regarding regulatory compliance. From this a list of suitable providers whose offerings are considered fit for purpose is prepared. At this stage the list should keep the options open, for example between laboratory and point-of-care provision, until a *'comparision of costs and features'* is made. There then follows *'negotiation and purchase'*. An acceptance procedure needs to be agreed with the manufacturer before an order is finally placed so any disputes over fitness for purpose can be resolved against a background of an objective specification. A partially completed IVD procurement form, in use at St Elsewhere's for a trial period, is shown in Figure 8.6.

IVD PROCUREMENT FORM

RECORD FILENAME	*MF-BIO-IVDPrc#Myocard Z*

1 Department	**2 Project name**
Biochemistry	*Measurement of Myocard Z*
4 Date project commenced	**5 Date project finished**
03/01/2002	

6 Assessment of need

The need to measure Myocard Z in plasma of ? myocardial infarction patients has been identified. A single measurement, 4 hours after the onset of chest pain has been shown to reliably identify those patients who can be safely discharged to the care of their primary care physicians without an overnight stay. Maximum benefit to the patient and to the working of the A & E department, requires results available 20 minutes after the sample has been taken. Recent installation of an air tube transport system allows tests to be performed in the laboratory on a 24 hour basis using existing equipment or a new dedicated analyzer. POCT in A & E is an option providing the available device is reliable and easy to use.

7 Market survey

No	Name of manufacturer	Name of IVD	Commentary
1	*Kyoto Diagnostics*	*BMH Analyser*	*New reagents for use on existing analyzer/laboratory*
2	*First Generation plc*	*MyoProfile 2002*	*Standalone instrument measuring Myocard Z (plus an option of two other tests out of three).*
3	*Venture BioScience Ltd*	*MyocardCARD*	*Single use POCT device*
4	*Dionysis Systems*	*MyoCardSTAT*	*Single use POCT device with built in internal quality control*

Figure 8.6 Procurement of IVDs form [MF-GEN-IVDPrc]

8 Collection of data (this includes all attached papers)

8.1 Financial comparison (initial figures in £ Sterling based on 2500 tests per annum)

No	Name of manufacturer/ IVD	Capital cost average per year over 5 yrs	Installation and training	Reagent cost/ test (including controls)	Staffing cost/ test
1	Kyoto Diagnostic/ BMH Analyzer	Existing equipment	Minimal	£ 1.30	Minimal
2	First Generation plc/ MyoProfile 2002	£ 1200.00	Training course including expenses £ 315.00	£ 3.45	To be determined
3	Venture BioScience Ltd/ MyocardCARD	Nil	Minimal	£ 12.65	To be determined

8.2 Checklist of other data

No	Name of manufacturer/ IVD	Manufacturer's performance claims	Evaluation reports	User experience	Regulatory compliance
1	Kyoto Diagnostic/ BMH Analyzer	Attached	To be available 01/03/2002	BMH Analyzer Users Group (3 users)	CE marked
2	First Generation plc/ MyoProfile 2002	Attached	None at present	Figures for European users attached	CE marking being sought

Figure 8.6 continued Procurement of IVDs form [MF-GEN-IVDPrc]

INSTRUCTIONS FOR USE

'Ideal Standard' clause 6.4.2 Instructions for use

As the concept of an IVD (Figure 8.1) goes far beyond that of an instrument or piece of apparatus or equipment, so the concept of 'instructions for use' is broadened. Clear instructions have a vital role in the provision of a quality service and attention to their content and quality is an integral part of a quality management system. The IVD Directive places a requirement on the manufacturer to supply appropriate instructions for use. If a user changes the intended use of an IVD with CE marking, or modifies the instructions for use without the agreement of the manufacturer, the user becomes liable for any resultant failure of performance.

It follows from this, therefore, that if a laboratory is preparing any laboratory procedures (commonly known as Standard Operating Procedures, SOPs) that give instructions for use, they must **exactly reproduce the manufacturer's**

instructions for how the device should be used, and all existing copies must be updated as appropriate (Chapter 5). In practice, laboratories do create laboratory procedures (SOPs) for their own use and this in the past has been occasioned by the poor quality of the information (e.g. a poor translation) provided by the manufacturer. Clearly dialogue between manufacturers organizations such as the European Diagnostics Manufacturers Association (EDMA), governmental agencies such as the Medical Devices Agency in the UK, and the users (through professional bodies such as the European Communities Committee for Clinical Chemistry EC4), can be a channel for continual improvement in this area.

In Chapter 10, further practical advice is given on how to deal with this situation in a cost effective and practical manner. All such instructions, whether they exist in hard copy or in electronic form, must be treated as controlled documents and all users must be aware of the current version of instructions for use, in particular staff in an on-call situation. The MDA-DB-IVDs points out that 'in the event of litigation by the patient or their representative, user organizations may need to call upon evidence that instructions were given to users in respect of equipment and upon documentary evidence that crucial steps in the process were, in practice, carried out'. This means that the manufacturer should have, and be kept informed of, users contact details so that updates are automatically sent.

The implementation of the IVD Directive has required the production of a number of European Standards and the task for their production has been assigned to the IVD committee of the European Committee for Standardization (CEN/TC 140). Certain of these standards are important to a laboratory wishing to judge the quality of information provided by the manufacturer and examples of this are EN 591:2001 'Instructions for in vitro diagnostic instruments for professional use' and EN 375:2001 'Information supplied by the manufacturer with in vitro diagnostic reagents for professional use' (see Figure 10.7 for contents). EN 591:2001 includes a recommended content of a user manual, the headlines of which are given in Figure 8.7. This recommended content shows a bias towards measuring equipment, but it could very easily be adapted to other equipment, such as staining machines or microtomes in histopathology or to a plate pouring machine in microbiology. It provides a good framework against which to judge users manuals to ensure that they contain all the information required. Similarly EN 375:2001 provides a basis with which to judge the quality of labelling of the outer container and the immediate container, and instructions for use for reagents. A parallel pair of standards EN 592:2001 and EN 376:2002 provide requirements for self testing devices.

0	TABLE OF CONTENTS	12	PRESENTATION OF ANALYTICAL DATA
1	GRAPHIC SYMBOLS	13	SPECIAL FUNCTIONS
2	MANUFACTURER	14	SHUT-DOWN PROCEDURE
3	IDENTIFICATION	15	EMERGENCY PROCEDURE
4	WARNINGS AND PRECAUTIONS	16	INTERNAL QUALITY CONTROL
5	INTENDED PURPOSE	17	DISPOSAL INFORMATION
6	INSTALLATION	18	MAINTENANCE
	6.1 General	19	TROUBLESHOOTING
	6.2 Action upon delivery	20	TECHNICAL SPECIFICATIONS
	6.3 Preparation prior to installation	21	DATE OF ISSUE OR REVISION
	6.4 Bringing into operation	22	SUPPLEMENTARY INFORMATION
7	THEORY		22.1 Brief operating instructions
8	FUNCTIONS		22.2 Lists of uses and applications
9	PERFORMANCE AND LIMITATIONS OF USE		22.3 Warranty information
			22.4 Ordering information
10	PREPARATION PRIOR TO USE		22.5 Possibilities of extension
11	OPERATING PROCEDURE		22.6 Assistance
			22.7 Supplementary theoretical information

based on EN 591:2001 'Instructions for in vitro diagnostic instruments for professional use'

Figure 8.7 Requirements for the content of a User Manual

TRAINING

'Ideal Standard' clause 6.4.3 Training

For CE marked IVDs, the IVD Directive stipulates as an 'essential requirement' that the obligation to provide proper training lies with the manufacturer. Proper training is an essential part of the introduction of any IVD and the importance of following the instructions is stressed in the previous section. A list of other considerations is given in Figure 8.8 and these need to be used in the setting of quality objectives and plans and in the annual joint review of staff (Figure 6.11). At St Elsewhere's records of all training and associated competence assessments are kept in the individual's training record (Figure 6.17).

An approach to **training staff in the use of** *in vitro* **diagnostic medical devices** should consider...

- which individuals within the laboratory (out of the total number who will be working with the IVD) should receive training offered by the manufacturer or supplier

- how the remaining individuals will be trained, by whom and the timescale

- when retraining is indicated

- training of temporary or locum staff

- training of out of hours (on-call) staff

- future training needs in the event that those trained directly by the manufacturer or supplier change jobs

- training in the event of instrument/software upgrades

based upon the MDA Device Bulletin 2002 (02)
'Management of *In Vitro* Diagnostic Medical Devices' 2002

Figure 8.8 Management of IVDs – Training

ACCEPTANCE TESTING, USER VERIFICATION AND VALIDATION
'Ideal Standard' clause 6.4.4 Acceptance testing, user verification and validation
In various published standards and guideline documents there is total confusion regarding the use of the terms verification and validation. Dictionaries of common English usage make no clear distinction between the two words and in published standards and guidelines they are used interchangeably. For the purposes of this book the starting place is with the ISO definitions shown in Figure 8.9.

Verification
Confirmation by examination and provision of objective evidence that specified requirements have been fulfilled

Validation
Confirmation by examination and provision of objective evidence that the particular requirements for a specific intended use are fulfilled

ISO 8402:1994 Quality management and quality assurance – Vocabulary

Figure 8.9 ISO definitions of verification and validation

These definitions are not easy to understand and are best explained with an example. If the laboratory orders an item, perhaps a new batch of internal quality control material, certain requirements will have been specified in the order, such as expiry date, bottle size, and target values for the analytes. User verification is checking upon receipt, to ascertain that 'what you get is what you ordered' by examining the labelling or package inserts. User validation requires using the material to see that the target values specified are within acceptable limits and it is therefore fit for its intended use.

Validation is demonstrated by manufacturer's data that support their performance claims. In ISO 9001:2000 this equates to activities described in clauses 7.3.6 *'Design and development validation'* and 7.3.7 *'Control of design and development claims'*. The IVD Directive requires that the manufacturer provides evidence in technical documentation that the IVD performs as claimed, whether these claims are of a technical, analytical or diagnostic nature. Such evidence can be shown by data already available to the manufacturer, by scientific literature or by data originating from performance evaluation studies in a clinical or other appropriate environment in accordance with the intended use. EN 13612:2002 'Performance evaluation of in vitro diagnostic medical devices' specifies the requirements for such studies. Such performance evaluation studies are often performed in co-operation with a user laboratory.

Whether all these activities are described in standards or guidelines as verification or as validation, they both have one objective and that is to ensure that an IVD used in an examination process is fit for that purpose. They are not a 'once only' activity in the laboratory; each new batch of internal quality control material is introduced into use via a separate verification and validation process.

The MDA-DB-IVDs, in the section on 'acceptance testing and user verification' suggests that there are three tests to be applied on delivery 'acceptance testing' which seems to equate with the ISO definition of verification; 'commissioning' which applies to complex instrumentation such as laboratory analyzers. This is often carried out by the supplier and the purpose is to ensure 'that it is in good and safe working order to be put into service'; and, 'user verification' which equates with the ISO definition of (user) validation in that it talks of 'the performance of the device'… being… 'comparable to the manufacturers claims' and fit for its intended use. It recommends comparing results with those from a previous methodology or being comparable with a gold standard.

In quality management terms, ISO 9001:2000 clause 7.5 *'Production and service provision'* (which is equivalent to pre-examination, examination and post-examination processes) says in the clause on validation that 'the organization shall demonstrate the ability of these processes to achieve planned results'. The aspect of validation of methods is dealt with in ISO 17025:1999 as a main clause, 5.4, *'Test (and calibration) methods and method validation'*. In ISO 15189:2002 clause 5.5, *'Examination procedures'* says with slightly less clarity 'the laboratory shall use only validated procedures to confirm that the examination procedures are suitable for intended use. The validations shall be as extensive as are necessary to meet the needs in the given field or field of application'. The issue of validation is dealt with in more detail in Chapter 10.

MAINTENANCE AND REPAIR
'Ideal Standard' clause 6.4.5 Maintenance and repair
Whether or not the equipment IVD inventory is held in a computer database or as hard copy, details of the maintenance contract and records of service visits, scheduled or unscheduled, can be kept in a linked computer file or on separate record sheets linked by a unique equipment code. In the case of large complex pieces of equipment requiring frequent user servicing, as well as scheduled and unscheduled maintenance, an alternative to keeping such information in the equipment inventory may be a hard copy or electronic record (log book) for each piece of equipment.

The record of maintenance or servicing should include when it was done, what was done, who did the work, and any record of testing/calibration/acceptance before being put back in use. Some documents required by the laboratory can end up in the accounts department of the host organization, but copies should be retained in the laboratory. If a backup instrument is used during the servicing, it is important to establish that the two instruments give comparable results. A log book may also be the chosen place in which to record calibration data, quality control and reagent changes, but the most effective arrangement has to be determined for each situation. The main objective, of maintenance and servicing records is to determine which equipment was in service on the day a particular examination was performed.

Before equipment is repaired or serviced on site or at the manufacturers, agent's or elsewhere it is important that, if appropriate, it should be decontaminated by suitably trained staff. Some manufacturers or suppliers require a 'Declaration of contamination status and authorization to work' before the engineer will commence work. The appropriate form [MF-GEN-IVDServ] for the Pathology Laboratory of St Elsewhere's Hospital Trust is shown in Figure 8.10 and is a form required by the procedure for procurement and management of equipment (Figure 8.5).

IVD SERVICING FORM
Contamination status and authorization to work

RECORD FILENAME	MF-GEN-IVDServ#IVD 006

1 Department	2 IVD name and model
Biochemistry	BHM Analyzer
3 IVD Inventory number	**4 Date**
IVD 006	7 May 2001

5 Record of procedure	Tick where appropriate
5.1 This equipment/item has not been used in an invasive procedure or been in contact with blood, other body fluids or pathological samples. It has been cleaned in preparation for inspection, servicing or repair.	☐
5.2 This equipment/item has been cleaned and decontaminated. The method of decontamination was:	☐
5.3 This equipment/item has not been decontaminated. The nature of the hazard and safety precautions to be adopted are:	☐

I declare that I have taken all reasonable steps to ensure the accuracy of the above information.

Authorized signature...Name(printed)...

Position ....Hospital and Department...

Tel/Bleep No...Date...

The hazards of working on this equipment/item have been explained to me and I agree to work within the guidelines

Signature...Name(printed)...

Company...Date...

Figure 8.10 Form for declaration of contamination status and authorization to work [MF-GEN-IVDServ]

ADVERSE INCIDENT REPORTING
'Ideal Standard' clause 6.4.6 Adverse incident reporting

Adverse incidents have been defined as 'incidents which produce, or have the potential to produce, unwanted effects involving the safety of patients, users and others'. The Pathology Laboratory at St Elsewhere's regards adverse incident reporting as an important priority, having had a major incident in the past in which excess stearic acid on polystyrene granules in collection tubes had caused falsely low calcium results by chelating ultrafilterable calcium in the patients samples. The procurement and management procedure used in the laboratory at St Elsewhere's (Figure 8.5) requires both internal reporting using a form [MF-GEN-IVDRep] and external notification via an on-line reporting facility (www.medicaldevices.gov.uk) or on a form [MF-GEN-AdvIncd] based upon the example provided in Appendix 3 of MDA-DB-IVDs (Figure 8.11). There is a legal requirements for manufacturers of medical devices with CE marking to report incidents to a Competent Authority (MDA in the UK) if they have the potential to cause death or injury to a patient, user or third party. For *users* of medical devices, although there is no legal requirement to report, the MDA strongly encourages the reporting of all adverse incidents. In the UK, an interesting development is the reporting system developed at Keele University by the Control Assurance Unit (CASU) and the Medical Devices Management Standard (www.casu.org.uk).

ADVERSE INCIDENT FORM

Origin of report:

The Director of the Pathology Laboratory,   Telephone (0800) 100200
St Elsewhere's Hospital Trust,   FAX (0800) 300400
Eastside Street, ST ELSEWHERE,   email   director@path-lab-st elsewhere.uk
East Loanshire, EL7 5XX

This report confirms a telephone report ☐   **a fax report** ☐   **neither** ☐

RECORD FILENAME	

1 Reporter		**2 Position**	
3 Department		**4 Date of report**	

5 Device description (tick one box only)

☐	Clinical Chemistry	☐	Microbiology	☐	Self/home testing
☐	Haematology	☐	Cytopathology/ Histopathology	☐	Genetic testing
☐	Immunology	☐	Extra-Lab Testing	☐	Specimen receptacle

6 Product

☐	Test kit - Colorimetric	☐	Instrumentation/	☐	Calibrators
☐	Test kit - Immunoassay		Software	☐	Reagent
☐	Test kit - Other	☐	QC materials	☐	Reagent strip

Figure 8.11 Adverse incident reporting form [MF-GEN-AdvIncd]

7 Details of the device - instrumentation		
Product name		
Model		
Manufacturer (including telephone no)		
Supplier (including telephone no)		
Serial No		Approximate age	
Is there a CE marking?	YES ☐　　　　NO ☐	

8 Details of the device - kits, reagents and specimen receptacles		
Brand name		
Analyte/Marker		
Manufacturer (including telephone no)		
Supplier (including telephone no)		
Batch No		Expiry date	
Is there a CE marking?	YES ☐　　　　NO ☐	

9 Nature of defect/details of incident

Contact name for further details		Telephone number	

10 Action taken by staff/manufacturer/supplier

Further details can be given on additional sheets if necessary.

Figure 8.11 continued Adverse incident reporting [MF-GEN-AdvIncd]

INVENTORY, STOCK CONTROL AND RECORDS

'Ideal Standard' clause 6.4.7 Inventory, stock control and records

A distinction was drawn earlier that the management of 'equipment IVDs' is through an equipment inventory and maintenance and repair records, whereas 'consumable IVDs', are managed through stock control mechanisms. The main purposes of equipment inventories, maintenance records and stock control are shown in Figure 8.12.

The purpose of keeping an **equipment inventory, maintenance records** and **stock control** is to...

- be able to audit whether a piece of equipment (IVD) was used at a particular time to carry out a particular examination process

- keep a record of maintenance contracts and servicing

- assist in replacement planning

Figure 8.12 Purposes of an equipment inventory

EQUIPMENT INVENTORY
Figure 8.13 shows the information required in an equipment inventory database. The unique inventory number for each piece of equipment can be cross-referenced to other documents, maintenance and repair records, calibration and safety records, manufacturer/supplier details and to manufacturer's handbooks, procedures/work instructions which describe how to use the equipment. If the equipment inventory is to be used for replacement planning, then additional information regarding the purchase price and scheduled replacement will need to be included.

CONSUMABLE IVDs AND STOCK CONTROL
There are two separate but inter-related issues concerning IVD consumables, reagents, calibration and quality control material. Firstly the management issues, i.e. the way they are procured (ordered, purchased, delivered), verified on receipt and stored prior to use, and secondly, the examination process activities, i.e. how they are issued, validated for use and their use recorded. At all stages in the cycle, records must be kept. On the management side this is important for stock control and financial management, and on the examination process side it is important in order to establish an audit trail which will allow the reconstruction of what consumables, reagents, calibration and quality control material were used when a particular batch of assays were performed.

These activities have to be part of a defined process which is illustrated in Figure 8.14 and are dependent on good stock control records. It is also necessary to either have an overall laboratory procedure for the validation and use of materials in examination processes, or to have clear instructions in the appropriate parts of any examination procedure which uses such material (Chapter 10).

Equipment identificatio n (Q-pulse terms)	Data entered
Data based identification (instrument number)	IVD0006
IVD general type (instrument description/type)	Analyze r
IVD Name and model	BHM Analyze r
Hospita l serial number(serial number)	SEHT-PATH- 9786
Department (department)	Pathology/Biochemistry
Location (location)	Room BIO-098
IV D procurement reference	MF-GEN-IVDPror # (system not in place at time of acquisition)
Date of purchas e	03/03/1999
Limitation of use (limitation of use)	Patholog y Laborator y
Link to current procedures	LP-BIO- BHMAnal z / LP-BIO- BHMMan
Link to manufacturer/supplier details (Q-pulse terms)	Data entered
Manufacturer/supplier name (supplier)	Kyoto Diagnostics
Addres s (address)	10 Linden Drive, Georgetown, Middleshire, UK
Te lephone (tel)	0298 67543
Fax (fax)	0298 67543
Emai l (Email)	Kyoto@aol.com
Contact name (contact)	Linda Brown (Technical support)
Link to maintenance and repai r records that include...	
Date in servic e - Date removed from servic e - disposal date - maintenanc e intervals - frequenc y of service	
Wa rranty details	
Maintenance and repair date s - damage, modification, malfunction or repair details - action taken - costs	
Link to financial and planning information...	
Cost information including initial purchas e price and if possible all ongoing maintenance, consumable and reagent cost s - p roposed replacement date	
Links to calibration and safet y r ecords can also be made in Q-pulse	

Figure 8.13 Contents of an equipment IVD inventory

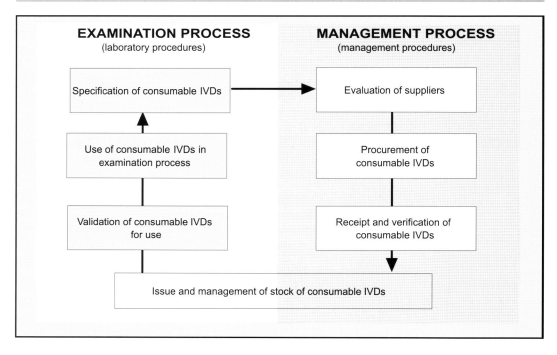

Figure 8.14 Management and use of consumable IVDs

Data items held in the stock control system at St Elsewhere's laboratory are shown in Figure 8.15.

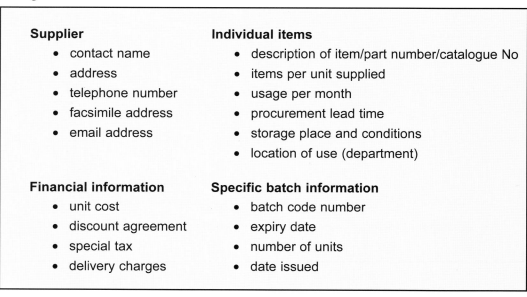

Figure 8.15 Data items for stock control system of consumable IVDs

MANAGEMENT OF DATA AND INFORMATION SYSTEMS

'Ideal Standard' clause 6.5 Management of data and information systems

Whilst computers are used very extensively in many pathology laboratories, not all data and information is managed using computers. However, the general principles are the same and concern the integrity, confidentiality and security of data and information. Examples of the use of computer systems are shown in Figure 8.16. Laboratory information systems (LIS) are central to the operation of many laboratories. Much of what is said in this section, whilst focusing on the management of such systems, will apply equally to other computer systems in the laboratory. Typically a LIS will not only capture, process, report and store data concerning the identification of patients and specimen analysis, but will also be able to communicate the results back to the requesting doctor. Automated laboratory equipment is controlled by computers, and the software which comes with these computers can prove more of a problem in the early evaluation than do mechanical functions of the equipment. The use of personal computers in the laboratory is now extensive and includes the creation and management of laboratory documentation, and the use of costing and financial management programmes.

- communication between the requester and the laboratory

- acquisition, processing, reporting and storage of data

- evaluation and presentation of quality control and quality assessment data

- operation and control of semi-automated and automated equipment

- direct/indirect capture of data from automated equipment

- matching of sample and library data

- performance of statistical functions

- creation and management of laboratory documentation

- monitoring and control of inventories

- stock control of reagents, consumables and standard material

- costing and financial management programmes

Figure 8.16 Uses of computers in the pathology laboratory

The requirements of International Standards regarding control of documentation and records has been discussed in Chapter 5, but other more technical issues concern the security, integrity, validation and management of data and are found in isolated clauses throughout the standards. The exception is ISO 15189:2002 which has an informative Annex B, 'Laboratory Information Systems'. The structure of clause 6.5 of the 'Ideal Standard' entitled 'Management of data and information systems' shown in Figure 8.17 is based upon Annex B and upon the OECD consensus document entitled 'The application of the principles of GLP to computerised systems'.

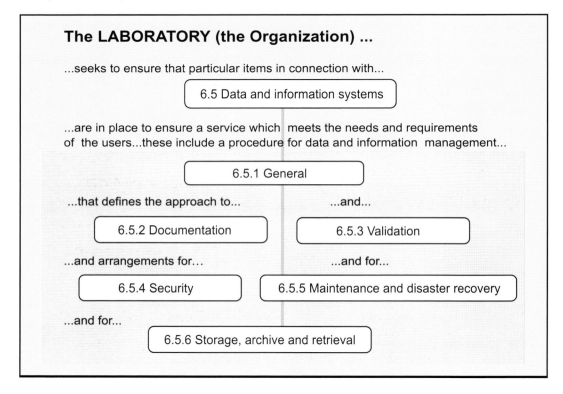

Figure 8.17 Clause 6.5 of the 'Ideal Standard' – Management of data and information systems.

GENERAL
'Ideal Standard' clause 6.5.1 General requirements
In the Pathology Laboratory of St Elsewhere's Hospital Trust the main day to day responsibility for running the laboratory computer is carried by the Computer Manager, who reports to the Business Manager. The Director of the Laboratory has overall responsibility for the management arrangements, but delegates this responsibility to a suitably experienced colleague, who acts as chairman of the

Laboratory Computer Working Group. The Computer Manager acts as secretary to the working group, and other members include the departmental database co-ordinators and representatives of other users, e.g. clerical staff. The database co-ordinators are appropriately trained laboratory staff who work closely with the Computer Manager to ensure that changes in hardware, software and database information are carried out in a structured, documented and reliable fashion. The contents of the procedure for the management of all data and information [MP-GEN-DataMan] within the the laboratory and at its interfaces with the users is shown in Figure 8.18. Particular aspects of this procedure are discussed briefly in the rest of the chapter, but it is important to remember that procurement and management of the purchase of computer systems is under the control of the procedure for management of IVDs, [MP-GEN-IVDPrc] (Figure 8.5).

---

0   INTRODUCTION

    0.1 Purpose and scope

    0.2 Responsibility

    0.3 References

    0.4 Definitions

    0.5 Documentation

1   ORGANIZATION AND MANAGEMENT

    1.1 Laboratory Computer Working
        Group

    1.2 Business Manager/Computer
        Manager

    1.3 Departmental database co-ordinators

2   DOCUMENTATION

    2.1 Procedure manuals

    2.2 Hardware inventory

    2.3 Communication inventory

    2.4 Software inventory including licences

    2.5 Software application descriptions

3   VALIDATION

    3.1 Acceptance

    3.2 Change control/configuration
        management

4   SECURITY

    4.1 Physical security

    4.2 Logical security

    4.3 Data integrity

    4.4 Backup

5   MAINTENANCE AND DISASTER RECOVERY

    5.1 Maintenance contracts for
        prevention and fault repair

    5.2 System disaster recovery plan

    5.3 Contingency plan

    5.4 Environmental control

6   ARCHIVING AND RETRIEVAL

    6.1 Archiving

    6.2 Archiving indexing

    6.3 Archive storage (including
        environmental control)

    6.4 Archive disposal

Figure 8.18 Contents of a procedure for the management of data and information [MP-GEN-DataMan]

All staff who have to use the computer, for whatever task, should be given adequate training. If they have access to the administration and configuration modules it is better if the original supplier trains them. With regard to software for personal computers, there are a number of companies who will arrange the training of staff on an off-site or on-site basis. Although the initial expenditure may seem large, it is worthwhile in the long term to ensure that training is done properly, because many software packages are in practice only utilised to some 20% of their capacity.

In some countries it is mandatory that any computer system which holds information concerning individual patients or members of staff must be registered under data protection legislation (for further discussion see under 'Security'). Under this legislation it is not only important that the computer facilities should be registered, but also that procedures are in place to enable information regarding individuals to be readily accessible upon request.

VALIDATION
'Ideal Standard' clause 6.5.2 Validation

As with any piece of equipment, procedures should be in place governing the acceptance of computer systems and their validation. A pragmatic definition of computer validation is provided in Figure 8.19 and the extent of validation required will depend on the type of hardware and software products involved.

Computer validation

Computers whatever their type, suffer from the "black-box" syndrome; an input is made at one end, an answer is produced at the other. Because what happens inside cannot be seen, it must be assumed that the box is functioning correctly. For the purposes of validation it is usually acceptable to assume correct operation if the computer produces expected answers when input with well-characterised parameters.

The degree of validation necessary depends on the exact use of the computer. For each computer the proposed use should be defined so that the degree of validation necessary may be established.

from Accreditation for Chemical Laboratories, EURACHEM Guidance document No.1/
WELAC Guidance Document No. WGD 2

Figure 8.19 Definition of computer validation

A note to sub-clause 5.4.7 in ISO 17025:1999, states that 'commercial off-the-shelf (e.g. word processing, database and statistical programmes) in general use within their designed application range may be considered to be sufficiently validated...' In a practical guide to the complex issue of 'Software Validation in Accredited

Laboratories' available at www.fasor.com. The author distinguishes commercial off-the-shelf software (COTS), from modified off-the-shelf software (MOTS), such as generic data acquisition software, the purchased portion of which can be regarded as COTS, but says that the modified part must be regarded as custom software (CUSTOM). CUSTOM software is code that is laboratory or sub-contractor written and should have evidence of validation. Details of validation beyond the pragmatic definition in Figure 8.19 are outside the scope of this book.

However, the key to successful validation is not to regard it as a static phenom-enon, but as an ongoing exercise sometimes termed 'configuration management' or 'change control'. It has been defined as 'a set of procedures that when followed, ensure adequate control, visibility and security of the version number, issue, and any changes made to hardware programme source codes, executable object codes, firmware, data, and electronic representation of documents. The procedures require that any modifications made, as well as the personnel making them, be authorized. The details of such changes shall be correctly recorded, together with details and results of tests carried out to validate the modified computer system'. This crucial activity ensures that all changes to software/hardware configurations are controlled and documented. It is important to distinguish between a software product and a computer system. A computer system being defined as the deployed software and hardware bundle. This is important because one software product can be deployed on a number of computer systems, i.e. versions of Microsoft Word. Some practical ideas to good software practices that will assist in managing validation and in ongoing quality management and data security are presented in Figure 8.20.

- treat each software product as a piece of equipment that has to be 're-calibrated' each time it is changed or modified

- place software products in a read only directory

- network computers so that they access a shared program on a server

- lock spreadsheet cells that contain mathematical computations

- password protect configuration files or set up screens

- backup, backup and backup off-site!

- plan for hardware/software recovery

based on Software Validation in Accredited Laboratories, A Practical Guide, GD Gogates 2001

Figure 8.20 Good practices in software management

At St Elsewhere's configuration management requires formal approval and documentation of any change to a computerised system. The Computer Manager has the responsibility for maintaining such records, and it is important that the Computer Manager works in close conjunction with people appointed as departmental database co-ordinators. In particular, changes might require training or retraining of staff, which should be recorded in the staff training record.

SECURITY
'Ideal Standard' clause 6.5.3 Security

It is important that physical security measures are in place to restrict access to any computer equipment. This often means that the security of the whole pathology laboratory should be maintained, as not all equipment will be found in a particular 'computer room'. Logical security requires that the user needs to enter a unique electronic signature or password which not only allows the user to use the computer, but also defines the level of access. The user's level of access will relate to the type of responsibility and tasks they have to perform. As a rule an individual's access should be restricted to those functions which it is necessary for them to perform. For example, a member of the laboratory staff who is responsible for entering information from request forms and specimen labels will only require the level of access to enable them to perform these particular functions.

Two further methods are available to improve both security and the integrity of the computer audit trail (Who did what and when?). A user should have the ability to change their password regularly and be locked out of the system if they fail to do so within a certain time period. In addition, computer terminals should be set to log out after a short period of inactivity to prevent other users from undertaking unauthorized tasks by continuing a session opened by another user with different priorities. It is important, not only that people are given passwords, but also that they understand the importance of the maintenance of data integrity on the system, and this should be part of their training.

It is also important to appreciate that data or software which comes to the laboratory on any form of electronic medium should be checked for viruses before it is introduced into the system. This is an increasing problem for all computers, and they should be provided with the most recent virus detection programmes. Failure to do this can lead to the irretrievable loss of data. The procedure for preparing backup copies of all the software should be clearly delineated. This will include not only backup copies of the data files, but also of the operating and applications software. Some hospital computer systems include laboratory modules, and the computing facility of the laboratory may then be situated and maintained outside the pathology laboratory. It is important to ensure under these circumstances that the procedure for the management of the laboratory computer encompasses a clear description of these arrangements, and how they might affect the integrity of data.

One of the key issues regarding security and integrity of data concerns 'the protection of individuals with regard to the processing of personal data and on the free movement of such data'. In the UK, the British Medical Association has produced some interim guidelines on the security of clinical systems. In addition they have commissioned the development of a clinical information security policy, which sets out nine principles of data security (Figure 8.21) that are designed to uphold the principle of patient consent and to be independent of specific equipment. Although most LIS systems have mechanisms to prevent the entry of spurious data by delineating the range or type of acceptable values (e.g. dates into date fields or limits on the numerical range of an analytical result), there remain areas for human decision such as the merger of multiple patient records. In the latter situation it is important to have clear rules for merger, such as a match for forename, surname, date of birth and where possible a unique patient number e.g. a national identity number.

Figure 8.20 mentioned a number of good practices in software management for protecting data These practices are an implicit rather than explicit requirement in many sub-clauses of ISO 17025:1999 and ISO 15189:2002. Further practical tips have been described in a paper (see Appendix 2 Further reading), entitled, 'Excel 97 Security' and deals with techniques for protecting cells in spreadsheets and workbooks and maintaining a change history. Similar protection and change history recording can be given to Word documents through the File/Save as/Options, and File/Versions, functions.

MAINTENANCE AND DISASTER RECOVERY
'Ideal Standard' clause 6.5.4 Maintenance and disaster recovery
The increasing dependence of laboratories on the reliability of computer systems makes effective maintenance and disaster recovery crucial. It is important to have a preventative maintenance contract which not only covers the maintenance of the hardware of the computer, but also covers the maintenance of the integrity of the operating system and applications software. A further development of this arrangement is a 'facilities management' system where the computer is provided and run by a commercial concern for an annual fee. The actual installation can be in the laboratory or a remote site. Even with commercially available systems, a laboratory can become over dependent on one person to maintain the system and it is crucial that systems are properly documented, and that other staff are trained to cope with emergency breakdowns.

1) **Access control** - Each identifiable clinical record shall be marked with an access control list naming the people or groups of people who may read it and append data to it. The system shall prevent anyone not on the list from accessing the record in any way.

2) **Record opening** - A clinician may open a record with herself and the patient on the access control list. When a patient has been referred she may open a record with herself, the patient, and the referring clinician(s) on the access control list.

3) **Control** - One of the clinicians on the access control list must be marked as being responsible. Only she may change the access control list and she may add only other health professionals to it.

4) **Consent and notification** - The responsible clinician must notify the patient of the names on his record's access control list when it is opened, of all subsequent additions and whenever responsibility is transferred. His consent must also be obtained, except in emergency or in a state of statutory exemptions.

5) **Persistence** - No one shall have the ability to delete clinical information until the appropriate time has expired.

6) **Attribution** - All accesses to clinical records shall be marked on the record with the name of the person accessing the record as well as the date and time. An audit trail must be kept of all deletions.

7) **Information flow** - Information derived from record A may be appended to record B, if and only if, B's access control list is contained in A's.

8) **Aggregation control** - Effective measures should exist to prevent the aggregation of personal health information. In particular, patients must receive special notification if any person whom it is proposed to add to their access control list already has access to personal health information on a large number of people.

9) **Trusted computer base** - Computer systems that handle personal health information shall have a sub-system that enforces the above principles in an effective way. Its effectiveness shall be evaluated by independent experts.

Anderson R, Clinical system security: interim guidelines Brit Med J 1996; 312 109-11

Figure 8.21 Nine principles of data security

Procedures need to be in place which deal with the partial or total failure of any computer system. When a piece of automated equipment is controlled by a computer, this can cause particular problems if the computer fails as it is impossible to decontaminate the equipment without a functioning computer. For this reason a clause is included in the IVD servicing form (Figure 8.10) where Section C states 'This equipment/item has not been decontaminated and the nature and risk of the safety precautions to be adopted are ....'. Procedures need to be in place that will not only result in the recovery of the computerised system but include mechanisms for ensuring the integrity of the data recovered. Should the 'down time' be extensive, then plans need to be well documented for the continuing provision of service, particularly in relation to work done on emergency specimens.

STORAGE, ARCHIVE AND RETRIEVAL
'Ideal Standard' clause 6.5.5 Storage, archive and retrieval
Even with large computers, there is a practical limitation on the amount of data that can be stored on line. Theoretically there should be no such limitation, and all data should be instantly available. However, it is often uneconomic to maintain all data on the system. It is therefore necessary to delineate an archiving policy and determine which particular item in a record will trigger an archive. In pathology laboratory systems the archiving is often triggered by a certain period of inactivity on the patient's record, such that if a patient has not presented for further work in the laboratory for two years their records are then archived.

It is important that any system of archiving has a system of indexing which will enable practical retrieval. Archiving is done on some form of electronic media, and the storage of these disks or tapes should be subject to proper conditions of environmental control so that they cannot suffer damage and loss. It may be necessary to dispose of archive material, but this must not be done without authorization at the level of the Director of Pathology or the Head of Department. Arrangements will need to be made for short term and long term access to archived material. Short term access does not normally constitute a problem as a disk or tape can be reloaded on the system and searched in a reasonably convenient manner. However, if it is intended that there should be long term storage of archived material, it may be that the computer system has changed both in terms of hardware and software. In this situation, thought will be needed about long term storage of the data and of the operating and applications software to enable retrieval of the data should a suitable computer platform still be available. Archived material and at least one copy of current backup material should be stored in a secure location, separate from the computer room and preferably separate from the laboratory.

DOCUMENTATION
'Ideal Standard' clause 6.5.6 Documentation
Computer documentation can be divided into user documentation, that provides information on the day to day use of the system, and documentation associated with maintenance tasks and configuration management, security and archiving activities. User documentation can be on line or as hard copy and many software products have extensive help functions. Unfortunately user manuals are more often written for the technically minded and not for the day to day user.

The computer hardware, like any other piece of equipment in the laboratory, should be subject to the procedure for management of equipment described in Chapter 7, including a record in the equipment inventory.

In addition, however, certain quality and accreditation systems require that details of applications running on the hardware should be kept. This is best done as a record on a separate form in a manual system or as a separate file in a relational database linked to the main file in the equipment inventory system through a unique number in both files. The OECD Environmental Monograph, No 116, 'The application of the principles of GLP to computerised systems' provides useful information (Figure 8.22).

For each application there should be documentation fully describing...

- The name of the application software or identification code and a detailed and clear description of the purpose of the application.

- The hardware (with model numbers) on which the application software operates.

- The operating system and other system software (e.g. tools) used in conjunction with the application.

- The application programming language(s) and/or database tools used.

- The major functions performed by the application.

- An overview of the type and flow of data/data design associated with the application.

- File structures, error and alarm messages, and algorithms associated with the application.

- The application software components with version numbers.

- Configuration and communication links among application modules and to equipment and other systems.

from Section 8 Documentation in 'The application of the principles of GLP to computerised systems'
Environmental Monograph No. 116 OECD Paris 1995

Figure 8.22 OECD-GLP requirements for application description

Chapter 9

Pre- and post-examination processes

INTRODUCTION
'Ideal Standard' clause 7 Examination processes

DEFINITIONS
This section is intended to serve as an introduction to this chapter and to Chapter 10 on examination processes. The use of the term 'examination', which is defined in ISO 15189:2002 as a 'set of operations having the object of determining a property', does not provide much enlightenment to the general reader. However, the note attached to the definition is more helpful, 'in some disciplines (e.g. microbiology) an examination is the total activity of a number of tests, observations or measurements'. This definition therefore encompasses, the analysis of a blood sample for glucose, the microscopic examination of a colony on an agar plate or of a liver biopsy. ISO 15189:2002 also recognises the concept of pre- and post-examination activities (equivalent to pre- and post-analytical activity) and in defining them makes clear the sequence of events familiar to all laboratory personnel.

---

pre-examination process

steps starting in chronological order from the clinician's request, including the examination requisition, preparation of the patient, collection of the primary sample, transportation to and within the laboratory and ending when the (analytical) examination starts

post-examination process

processes following the examination, including systematic review, formatting and interpretation, authorization for release, reporting of results, transmission of results and storage of the samples of the examinations

ISO 15189:2002 Medical laboratories - Particular requirements for quality and competence

---

Figure 9.1 ISO 15189:2002 definitions of pre- and post-examination processes

REQUIREMENTS
The relationships between clauses of ISO 17025:1999 and ISO 15189:2002 and pre-examination, examination and post-examination processes are not easy to discern

from the headings of the clauses or from their arrangement within the Standards. In order to prevent repetition in the text and for ease of reference, in Figure 9.2, the clauses containing relevant material are grouped against the pre-examination, examination and post-examination clauses of the 'Ideal Standard'. Appendix 1 gives these relationships in more detail.

The 'Ideal Standard	ISO 17025:1999	ISO 15189:2002
7.1 Pre-examination processes	4.7 Service to the client	4.7 Advisory services
	5.7 Sampling	5.4 Pre-examination procedures
	5.8 Handling test and calibration procedures	
7.2 Examination process	5.4 Test and calibration methods and method validation	5.5 Examination processes
	5.6 Measurement traceability	
	5.9 Assuring the quality of test and calibration items	5.6 Assuring the quality of examinations
	4.9 Control of nonconforming testing and/or calibration work	4.9 Identification and control of nonconformities
7.3 Post-examination	4.9 Control of nonconforming testing and/or calibration work	4.9 Identification and control of nonconformities
	4.7 Service to the client	4.7 Advisory services
	5.10 Reporting results	5.7 Post-examination
		5.8 Reporting of results

Figure 9.2 Relationships between the pre-examination, examination and post-examination clauses of the 'Ideal Standard' and ISO 17025:1999 and ISO 15189:2002

Figure 9.3 shows the sub-clauses of clause 7 of the 'Ideal Standard' and their inter-relationships. This arrangement is based upon the current version of CPA(UK)Ltd, 'Standards for the Medical Laboratory'.

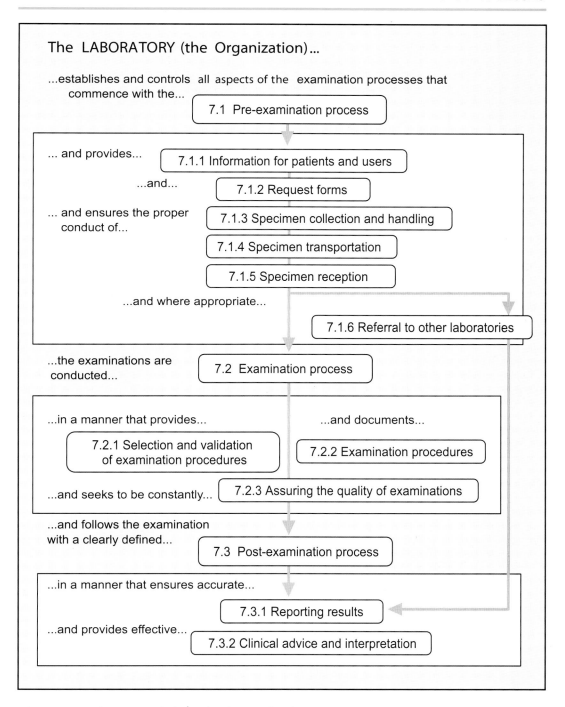

Figure 9.3 Clause 7 of the 'Ideal Standard' – Examination processes

EFFECTIVE PLANNING

A major task in preparing a laboratory to operate in conformance with standards is the creation of the procedures and other documentation that are required to describe and document pre-examination, examination and post-examination processes. It is very important to decide on what documentation is required at an early stage. At this point a quick reference back to Figures 3.10 and 5.3 will remind the reader of the 'sequence of action in quality management' and the hierarchy of documentation required to implement this sequence.

All documentation created should have a useful purpose and particularly in relation to examination procedures it is very important to utilise material provided by manufacturers in order to save time and effort and to avoid 're-inventing the wheel' (Chapter 10).

The approach at St Elsewhere's was to consider pre-examination, examination and post-examination processes across the whole of the Pathology Laboratory. These were then mapped using the logical order of the clauses of the 'Ideal Standard' and annotated with the informative filenames of the documents required. Figure 9.4 shows the diagram created, which forms an important part of the Quality Manual. It does not show the detail of processes associated with the laboratory information system (LIS) and their relationship with the hospital information system (HIS) via order communications. At St Elsewhere's these are mapped as an overlay to Figure 9.4 and described in a practical procedure [LP-GEN-LISHbk], called the Laboratory Information System Handbook.

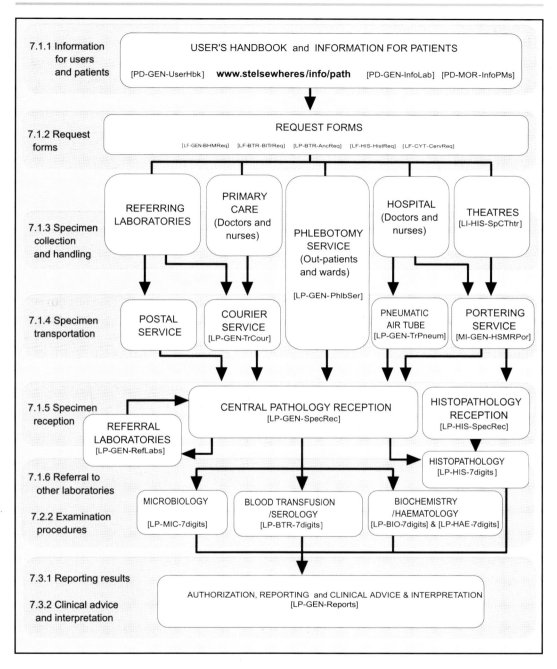

Figure 9.4 Pre-examination, examination and post-examination processes

PRE-EXAMINATION PROCESS
'Ideal Standard' clause 7.1 Pre examination process

In the pre-examination process, two key activities take place. Firstly, the formulation of a clinical question and the selection of the appropriate examinations, and secondly the practical steps of ordering, collection and handling, transportation and reception of samples prior to the examination itself. A central issue in these practical steps is maintaining the integrity of the relationship between the primary sample(s) taken from the patient and the patient, (did primary sample A, come from patient A?) between the primary sample(s) and the request documentation, (does request form A refer to primary sample A?) and then finally, in the preparation process, the relationship between the primary sample and secondary preparations from the primary sample (was blood film A prepared from primary sample A?). In forensic medicine these relationships are evocatively, but effectively, referred to as a 'chain of custody.

In ISO 15189:2002 clause 5.4 *'Pre-examination procedures'*, includes requirements for a request form, a primary sample collection manual, the traceability of primary samples to an identified individual (the patient), monitoring of samples in transport, recording of receipt of samples, processing of urgent samples and policies for rejection of samples. The requirements for the contents of a 'primary sample collection manual' as specified in ISO 15189:2002, whilst desirable, are difficult to reconcile in one document, as they require information for users, patients and laboratory processes to be included. However, the requirements are adequately covered at St Elsewhere's in a number of documents, including a users handbook [LP-GEN-UserHbk], a phlebotomy service procedure [LP-GEN-PhlbSer] and in some cases, information for patients, e.g. 'A guide to the laboratory' [PD-GEN-InfoLab], 'Information regarding post-mortems' [PD-MOR-InfoPMs], and 'A patient's guide to Diabetes' [PD-BIO-DiabGde] written in conjunction with the Department of Endocrinology.

INFORMATION FOR USERS AND PATIENTS
'Ideal Standard' clause 7.1.1 Information for users and patients

INFORMATION FOR USERS
The importance of the provision of consultant advice as part of a laboratory service is made clear in the description of a laboratory service given in Figure 3.1 and NPAAC Standard 2 'Staffing, supervision and consultation', which states that 'there shall be staff who can advise on the selection of tests, the evaluation and interpretation of laboratory results and the validity of the methods employed in the laboratory'. The way in which a doctor formulates the need for an examination or test and then chooses the correct examination will depend, firstly on the reason for the request, secondly on their training in the use of the laboratory, and

thirdly on the information provided by the laboratory.

There are a number of reasons why laboratory examinations are ordered (Figure 9.5) and all medical staff on arrival in the hospital, as part of their induction programme, should be provided with information on the use of the laboratory and encouraged to visit the laboratory to meet the senior staff. As junior medical staff have an enormous amount of information to digest in their first few days at a new hospital, the information needs to be presented in a clear and easily accessible format.

Laboratory examinations provide **information** to assist in the...

- Diagnosis of disease

- Screening for disease

- Determination of disease severity

- Determination of patient management

- Monitoring of disease progress

- Detection and monitoring of drug toxicity

- Prediction of response to treatment

Figure 9.5   Reasons for ordering laboratory examinations

As can be seen from Figure 9.6, at St Elsewhere's the laboratory still has the traditional User's Handbook (registered on Q-Pulse as a public document [PD-GEN-UserHbk]). However, the laboratory is now at the early stages of experimenting with the use of the hospital website (www.stelsewheres/info/path) as a source of laboratory and clinical information. The use of web technology for provision of information has a number of advantages, the information on the site can be regularly reviewed and each page of information can indicate the author and the review date. The provision of search facilities and the ability to move via hyperlinks from one part of the website to another, enable connections to be made that transcend departmental divisions. The traditional User's Handbook often presents information on a departmental basis, whereas in reality, questions arise in a different manner through the presentation of a clinical problem or from a query such as, 'how can I get Myocard Z measured? This query is not presented as 'in which department can I get Myocard Z measured?' and, therefore the ability to search by analyte or examination or clinical condition is more important than by department.

Web technology is not available to all and, therefore, a user's handbook will still be required by many laboratories. The content of the user's handbook is important, but its presentation is equally important and careful thought should be given to its design, size and durability. The first question to consider is whether it should be in the form of a bound booklet or loose leaf. The pro's and con's are difficult. A booklet in an A5 presentation is commonly used as it fits well into the outside pocket of a doctor's white coat, but used in these circumstances it will need a laminated cover to give it durability. The advantage of a loose leaf format, whether it is in an A5 binder or in the popular *'Filofax©'* format, is that updated pages can be issued. However, because of the numbers of copies of the user's handbook that have to be issued, the updates are not easy to control. On balance the bound format is probably easier to control as new editions can be circulated with a letter requesting the recipients to destroy their previously issued edition and perhaps with a return slip requiring acknowledgement of receipt.

The content of the handbook will depend to some extent on who the user is likely to be, e.g. handbooks for laboratories which are not directly connected to a hospital may not have a description of phlebotomy services to outpatients and hospital wards, but may need to describe the arrangements for the dispatch and receipt of specimens sent by air. The contents of the handbook currently in use at St Elsewhere's are shown in Figure 9.6.

The NPAAC publication, 'Guidelines for the preparation of laboratory manuals' first published in 1986 but reprinted in 1999, contains useful information on contents of a Laboratory Handbook. Laboratories (referral laboratories) that receive specimens from other laboratories require User Manuals, and good examples of these can be found on the website of the Public Health Laboratory Service, London, UK (www.phls.org.uk).

INFORMATION FOR PATIENTS
There are two specific issues concerning information for patients, firstly, how to access the services? and secondly the more difficult issue of ensuring that patients understand any procedures (e.g. phlebotomy) that are taking place and that they have given informed consent.

The first item of patient information at St Elsewhere's, is a three-fold general leaflet for patients visiting the laboratory [PD-GEN-InfoLab]. This is based on the approach described in Figure 7.8 and contains information on how to contact the laboratory and how to get there (bus routes etc.), a site map including details of parking and a brief description of the Pathology Laboratory and the services it offers. It is available at all primary care centres served by the laboratory and the site map it contains is also reproduced on the back of the general request form [LF-GEN-BHMReq] discussed below.

1 GENERAL INFORMATION
1.1 Postal address
1.2 Where to find us
1.3 Key personnel, their position and contact information
1.4 Population served
1.5 Laboratory hours

2 USE OF THE LABORATORY
2.1 Requests to the laboratory
- Requesting procedures (routine, urgent and out of hours)
- Completing the request form
- Patient identification and specimen collection
- Specimen labelling
- Specimen containers and where to get them
2.2 Collection of specimens (Phlebotomy service)
2.3 Transport to the laboratory
- Courier service
- Portering schedules
- Pneumatic air tube system
- Postal service
2.4 Results including method and times of reporting

3 OUT OF HOURS SERVICE
3.1 Examinations provided
3.2 Arrangements for interpretation and advice

4 BIOCHEMISTRY
4.1 Biochemistry mini-profiles
4.2 Information regarding dynamic function tests
4.3 Therapeutic drug monitoring
4.4 Storing specimens overnight
4.5 Urine and faecal collections - special instructions
4.6 Point-of-care testing

5 HAEMATOLOGY AND BLOOD TRANSFUSION
5.1 Haematology mini-profiles
5.2 Clotting studies
5.3 Bone marrow examination
5.4 In vivo investigations
5.5 Blood group (antenatal and transfusion)
5.6 Cross matching (routine and emergency)
5.7 Use of blood products (clinical procedures)
5.8 Transfusion reaction procedures

6 MICROBIOLOGY
6.1 Antibiotic service
6.2 Hospital infection
6.3 Blood cultures
6.4 Urine, faecal and seminal fluid

7 HISTOPATHOLOGY/CYTOPATHOLOGY
7.1 Surgical biopsies
7.2 Frozen section bookings
7.3 Requests for consented post-mortems
7.4 Coroner's post-mortems
7.5 Special requirements for samples, including cervical smears

8 ALPHABETICAL TABLES OF EXAMINATIONS

These tables are divided by department and contain the name of the test, specimen and container required, reference intervals (where appropriate), special comments and turnaround time.

Figure 9.6 Contents of pathology user's handbook [PD-GEN-UserHbk]

In certain situations there is need for more specific information to be available. Recent problems with retention of organs following post-mortems, particularly on children, have highlighted the need to provide good quality information to patients and their relatives. The Convention on Human Rights and Biomedicine promulgated by the Council of Europe includes a number of important Articles (Figure 9.7), which are quoted in recent advice from the Chief Medical Officer in the UK entitled, 'The Removal, Retention and use of Human Organs and tissue from Post-mortem Examinations'.

Article 2

'The interest and welfare of the human being shall prevail over the sole interest of society or science'

Article 5

'An intervention in the health field may only be carried out after the person concerned has given free and informed consent to it.

This person shall beforehand be given appropriate information as to the purpose and nature of the intervention as well as on its consequences and risks.

The person may freely withdraw consent at any time'

Article 22

'When in the course of an intervention any part of a human body is removed, it may be stored and used for a purpose other than that for which it was removed, only if this is done with appropriate information and consent procedures'.

Convention on Human Rights and Biomedicine, Council of Europe, European Treaty Series No 164, 1997

Figure 9.7 Articles of the Convention on Human Rights and Biomedicine

At St Elsewhere's, the pathologists seek to follow the articles of the Convention in their approach to post-mortems by offering relatives an advisory booklet (registered in Q-pulse as [PD-MOR-InfoPMs] when seeking consent to undertake a post-mortem examination. The content is based upon material prepared by the Royal College of Pathologists, 'Examination of the body after death, information about post-mortem examination for relatives' and upon an approach adopted by another Trust which uses the question and answer format as shown in Figure 9.8.

The latter approach was awarded a 'Clear English' Standard by the Plain Language Commission. A consent form is completed *with* the relative or representative which requires *explicit consent or otherwise* to: photography, the option of limited post-mortem, organs being taken or held, disposal of tissue blocks and of any tissue or organs taken and unlimited retention for purposes of medical research and education. A copy of the completed form is given to the relative or representative. In relation to phlebotomy the general rule is that formal consent is not required and that acceding to the procedure indicates implicit consent. This is, however, less clear in the case of a person unable to give formal consent or have a proper understanding of the situation. Consent to use specimens, other than tissues and organs, for purposes other than diagnosis is dealt with in the section on control of clinical material.

Patients who are required to undertake preparation for specific tests, or who have to undergo long term monitoring by the laboratory, are also provided with information. For example, for patients required to collect samples for semen analysis [PD-HAE-SemenCl] or patients undergoing long term monitoring of anticoagulant therapy [PD-HAE-AntiCoa].

The post-mortem
What is a post-mortem?
Who does the post-mortem?
Who can ask for a post-mortem?

Coroner's post-mortems
Why does the doctor contact the coroner?
Who carries out the post-mortem?
What about funeral arrangements?

Consented post-mortems
What does 'giving consent' mean?
-Full post-mortem
-Limited post-mortem

Other questions you may have
Where does the post-mortem take place?
When will the post-mortem take place and will it delay the funeral?
What happens during the examination?
Will the body be disfigured?
Do I have to consent to a post-mortem?
Will I find out the results of the post-mortem?

Keeping tissue, organs and body parts
Will the pathologist want to keep any tissue, organs or body parts after the post-mortem?
What is the stored material used for?
Photography and video recording
Do pathologists keep these items for a long time?
If I give the pathologist permission to keep tissue, organs or body parts, what will happen to them?
What if I give the pathologist my permission - and then change my mind?
Do I have to let you keep tissue, organs or body parts?
How will I know what tissue, organs or body parts you have kept?
Who do I contact if I need information before I decide what to do?

based on 'Examining the body after death - information for relatives about post-mortems' Chesterfield and North Derbyshire Royal Hospital NHS Trust.

Figure 9.8 Examining the body after death – information for relatives about post-mortems

REQUEST FORM
'Ideal Standard' clause 7.1.2 Request form

In a busy hospital, request forms (whether hard copy or electronic) from clinicians and the reports issued by the laboratory are a major means of communication, supplemented by a range of other opportunities that include clinico-pathological conferences, clinical audit meetings and, if time permits, a cup of coffee in the canteen!

In some countries the request form is called a requisition form. At the present time perhaps the majority of requests made by clinicians for examinations are made using a form. At St Elsewhere's computer terminals on the wards and in the emergency department enable requests to be made on the laboratory computer through an order communications system. In this case the patient's identification details are obtained from the patient master index of the hospital patient management system (PMS) or from the laboratory computer's patient database that is refreshed periodically by information from the PMS. This obviates the problems of transcribing the doctors handwriting and, in the case of hospital in-patients, ties the patient identification to what is hopefully, but not always reliably, a unique hospital number. For all other requests a thin card request form is used and can be regarded as the equivalent of a referral letter from one doctor to another. It is often the first step in a consultation between the requesting doctor and the laboratory. In order for the laboratory to undertake its tasks properly, the request form must be designed in a way which makes it easy for the requesting doctor to provide necessary information.

In ISO 15189:2002, clause 5.4.1 in the *'Pre-examination procedures'* section requires that the request form have space for the inclusion of certain items of information, but recognising that satisfactory clinical information is not always provided, does not make it obligatory upon the laboratory that *all* the information be collected. It is important when trying to motivate staff to carry out the rather monotonous task of data acquisition effectively, for the training to include instruction on the reasons for its collection and to involve staff in internal audits (see Chapter 11). Information is required for a number of specific purposes which are outlined in Figure 9.9. With the exception of a space to include the time and date of reception of the sample, all the items required by ISO 15189:2002 are included. If the laboratory is not computerised it can be useful to include a space for time and date of reception. Some laboratories have time and date stamp instruments to print this automatically on the request card. In an adequately staffed, well organized, and computerised laboratory, the time of arrival is almost the same as the time of accession.

Information	Reason
Patient's name Unit number Date of birth Sex	Identification and (age, sex) interpretation of results
Return address (e.g. ward, clinic, surgery telephone/pager number if urgent)	Delivery of report
Name of clinician (and telephone/pager number)	Liaison, auditing, billing
Clinical details (including drug treatment)	Justification of request Audit Interpretation Selection of appropriate tests Choice of analytical method (to avoid drug interference)
Test(s) required	Instruction to analyst
Sample(s) required	Instruction to phlebotomist
Date (and time if appropriate)	Identification Interpretation (with timed/sequential requests) Audit

based on Clinical Biochemistry, edited by Marshall WJ and Bangert SK, Churchill Livingstone 1995

Figure 9.9 Rationale for information required on a completed request form

There is a tendency in some laboratories to have a large number of specialised request forms for particular situations. However, the fewer request forms that are presented to the requesting doctor the easier it is for the necessary information to be provided. Increasing numbers of laboratories have a general form for the most common biochemistry, haematology and microbiology requests. An example of the general form [LF-GEN-BHMReq] used by St Elsewhere's Hospital Trust is shown in Figure 9.10. At St Elsewhere's, other request forms are restricted to blood transfusion, histopathology and cervical cytology.

St Elsewhere's Hospital Trust - **Pathology Laboratory**	Telephone (0800) 100200 Facsimile (0800) 300400 enquiries@pathlab-st elsewhere.uk
PATIENT NUMBER	LABORATORY ACCESSION NUMBER
SURNAME	REQUESTING DOCTOR (please print name) Signature
FORENAMES	Bleep number
ADDRESS	HOSPITAL WARD/CLINIC
	DATE & TIME OF COLLECTION
DATE OF BIRTH SEX male/female	
CONSULTANT/GENERAL PRACTITIONER (Name and number)	CLINICAL DETAILS/DIAGNOSIS/THERAPY

BIOCHEMISTRY		HAEMATOLOGY		MICROBIOLOGY		
☐ Renal profile	☐ Lipid profile	☐ Full blood count	☐ RA Latex	URINE	MSU	☐
☐ Liver profile	☐ Diabetic profile	☐ ESR	☐ Anti nuclear factor		CSU	☐
☐ Bone profile	☐ Fasting glucose	☐ B12 & folate	☐ Warfarin control (INR)	FAECES	Culture	☐
☐ Cardiac profile	☐ Random glucose	☐ Ferritin	☐ Coagulation screen		Parasites	☐
☐ Thyroid profile	☐ Pregnancy test	☐ IM screen	☐ Heparin control (APTT)	SPUTUM	Routine	☐
					AFB	☐
				SWAB	HVS	☐
					Urethral	☐
					Cervical	☐
Please specify other items		Please specify other items		Other from where CLOTTED BLOOD for................................		
				OTHER SPECIMEN for................................		

Figure 9.10   The general request form for biochemistry, haematology and microbiology [LF-GEN-BHMReq]

SPECIMEN COLLECTION AND HANDLING
'Ideal Standard' clause 7.1.3 Specimen collection and handling
There are three main elements to this step, proper identification of the patient from whom the sample is to be collected, its collection and, when appropriate, patient preparation.

IDENTIFICATION AND COLLECTION
The mechanism by which the specimen is associated with the patient and the request card is of utmost importance. When a pathology specimen is collected

from a patient, particularly outside hospital, it is unusual for unique identification labels for the specimen to be produced prior to, or at the time of, the specimen collection and heavy reliance has to be placed on the proper completion of the request form and the specimen container label. In some situations there are computer systems (described earlier) which allow the request to be made to the laboratory via a remote terminal. This is the situation with the phlebotomy service at St Elsewhere's where the LIS can prepare a phlebotomy work list with details of the patients' identity, their location in the hospital, and the investigations required. At the same time, unique identification label(s) are produced for attaching to the specimen container(s). In this situation the person collecting the sample has to positively identify the patient and collect the sample into the uniquely identified specimen container.

Hospital in-patients normally wear identification bracelets which must be checked carefully before the specimen is collected. This process could be the first step in what is called 'positive specimen identification'. This is where the identification data affixed to the specimen/container at source remains with that specimen throughout analysis, is read electronically by laboratory analyzers and computers and is printed on the final report without the need for any manual transcription. In order to reduce transcription errors to a minimum each specimen and the patient, who might have more than one specimen in the laboratory at any one time, have to be unequivocally identified.

More usually, however, a completed request card is received by the laboratory either with a specimen or in order to activate the phlebotomist or blood-taker into collecting the sample from the patient. At St Elsewhere's this is the case with specimens arriving from other hospitals (referring hospitals) or from primary care centres. It is important to ensure that certain minimum data is recorded on the specimen container and on the request card so that they can be unequivocally related. A minimum of information would be the name of the patient, date of birth, and the date of collection, preferably with some identification number relating to the hospital admission in the case of an in-patient.

In certain situations, particular care should be taken with regard to the adequacy of specimen collection, and in the case of cytopathology it is an important part of the receipt of the specimen that its adequacy should be determined. With many pathological specimens some of the most important sources of interference with the subsequent analysis can be associated with factors present at the time of sampling, and subsequent attempts to preserve or stabilise the specimens during transport or storage. In addition to communicating these issues through the User's Handbook at St Elsewhere's, the processes for the phlebotomy service are detailed in a procedure [LP-GEN-PhlbSer] and those for the specimen collection in operating theatres in [LP-HIS-SpCThtr] (Figure 9.4).

PATIENT PREPARATION
In addition to the collection and transportation of the sample, for certain biochemical and haematological tests it is important to standardize the preparation of the patient, e.g. fasting for sixteen hours for serum triglycerides, or be clear that the specimen has been collected at a specific time in relation to medication, e.g. therapeutic drug monitoring. Information concerning these issues should be included in the user handbook. Other clinical procedures [CP-], prepared in conjunction with the appropriate clinicians, should be provided by the laboratory and may include those for the collection of blood gases, conduct of glucose tolerance tests, and other dynamic function tests. If the procedure is novel or experimental then the approval of a local ethical committee must be sought.

SPECIMEN TRANSPORTATION
'Ideal Standard' clause 7.1.4 Specimen transportation
Figure 9.4 indicates that there are five distinct ways in which specimens are transported to and from the laboratory at St Elsewhere's. Specimens arrive and are dispatched by postal services, using a pneumatic air tube or via phlebotomists, and finally the courier and portering services. Each method presents its own problems, which fall into two categories; those associated with the arrival of the specimen in a fit condition for examination and those concerned with the health and safety of all personnel who might come into contact with the specimen, or its container, in transit. Both are in different ways, vitally dependent on the manner in which the specimen is transported. The contents of the World Health Organization (WHO), 'Guidelines for the Safe Transport of Infectious Substances and Diagnostic Specimens' are shown in Figure 9.11.

The document is intended to provide practical guidance to the section of the 'UN Recommendations on the Transport of Dangerous Goods' that deals with *diagnostic specimens* and *infectious substances*. International regulations promulgated by the Universal Postal Union (UPU) and the International Air Transport Association (IATA) are based upon this guidance. NPAAC's guideline on 'Information on the transport of pathology specimens' gives further detail on the IATA Dangerous Goods Regulations, 1998, good practical advice on 'the general principles of packaging' and an appendix which includes relevant extracts from the regulations.

- **Definitions**
  - Infectious substances
  - Diagnostic specimens

- **Packaging, Labelling and Documentation for Transport**
  - Basic Triple Packaging System
  - Requirements for Infectious Substances
  - Requirements for Diagnostic Specimens
  - Requirements for Air Mail
  - Refrigerants

- **Local Surface Transport**

- **Transport Planning**

based on Guidelines for the Safe Transport of Infectious Substances and Diagnostic Specimens
WHO/EMC/97.3 1997

Figure 9.11 WHO 'Guidelines for the Safe Transport of Infectious Substances and Diagnostic Specimens' – contents

From the point of view of the medical laboratory, the majority of specimens fall within the category, 'diagnostic specimens'. These are defined as 'any human or animal material including, but not limited to, excreta, blood and its components, tissue and body fluids, collected for the purposes of diagnosis, but excluding live infected animals' and 'specimens resulting from medical practice and research are considered a negligible threat to public health'. 'Infectious substances' are defined as 'a substance containing a viable microorganism, such as a bacterium, virus, rickettsia, parasite or fungus, that is known or reasonably believed to cause disease in humans or animals'. This definition does not include 'prions' although they are considered to be infectious agents. Included in the explanation to the definition of infectious substances are two situations of importance to the medical laboratory, a) those sample(s) from a patient with 'a serious disease of unknown cause' and, b) 'specimens….designated as infectious by a qualified person, e.g. a physician, scientist, nurse etc.'. The guidelines provide information on an approved triple packing system, the limits on amounts of material that can be sent in a primary container and include advice on the use of refrigerants.

POSTAL SERVICE
Requirements for air mail are given in the WHO Guidelines and most countries have their own regulations for packing and dispatch of diagnostic specimens.

Companies that produce materials for packing aim to meet these regulations.

COURIER AND PORTERING SERVICES

At St Elsewhere's, the courier and portering services are provided by a private company and are the subject of a formal contract. The principle of safe transport for these services is the same as for air or international transport; 'the material should not have any possibility of escaping from the package under normal conditions of transport'. The contract at St Elsewhere's is based upon the advice given in the WHO Guidelines in the section on local surface transport (Figure 9.12). The only exception being that the majority of primary containers are transported in plastic sealable bags that form an integral part of the request form. Where possible these are held upright in the transport box. Although the courier and portering services are provided by a private contractor, the regular cleaning and decontamination of the transport boxes is carried out in the central pathology reception area and the process is detailed in the appropriate procedure [LP-GEN-SpecRec] (Figure 9.14).

The following practices for **local surface transport** should be observed;

1. specimen containers should be watertight and leak-proof,

2. if the specimen container is a tube, it must be tightly capped and placed in a rack to maintain it in an upright position,

3. specimen containers and racks should be placed in robust, leak-proof plastic or metal transport boxes with secure, tight fitting covers,

4. the transport box should be secured in the transport vehicle,

5. each transport box should be labelled appropriately consistent with its contents,

6. specimen data forms and identification data should accompany each transport box,

7. a spill kit containing absorbent material; a chlorine disinfectant, a leak-proof waste disposal container and heavy duty reusable gloves should be kept in the transport vehicle.

NOTE: the practices 1-7 described above are not intended to supercede local or national requirements

based on Guidelines for the Safe Transport of Infectious Substances and Diagnostic Specimens
WHO/EMC/97.3 1997

Figure 9.12 WHO Guidelines – section on local surface transport

PNEUMATIC AIR TUBE

The HSE, (UK) have produced a useful information sheet that aims to provide guidance on the safe use of this method of transporting specimens (Figure 9.13), and is supplementary to the NHS Estates publication on the same topic entitled, 'Design Considerations, Good Practice Guide and Management Policy'. It draws attention to the fact that both the employer and employee using these systems will have duties under health and safety law, as all pathology specimens may contain substances that are hazardous to health and that others may contain hazardous chemicals, (e.g. specimens for histopathology in formalin solutions). It defines the areas of risk and focuses on risk control, suitability of specimen type, carrier design, specimen packing, spillage containment/clean up procedures and on information, instruction and training.

Introduction	**Suitability of specimen type**
Background	**Carrier design**
The law	**Specimen packing**
Assessing the risk	**Spillage containment/clean-up procedures**
Preventing and controlling the risk	**Information, instruction and training**

from HSE information sheet - Safe use of pneumatic air tube transport systems for pathology specimens

Figure 9.13   Safe use of pneumatic air tube transport systems for pathology specimens

SPECIMEN RECEPTION

'Ideal Standard' clause 7.1.5 Specimen reception

ISO 15189:2002 requires that 'all primary samples received shall be recorded in an accession book, worksheet, computer or comparable system' and that 'the date and time of receipt of samples, as well as the identity of the receiving officer, shall be recorded'. The arrangements in a pathology laboratory for specimen reception and data acquisition will vary according to how the laboratory is organized but these basic requirements can readily be met by a well thought out manual system or a LIS. In some hospitals, specimens go directly to the department concerned, or there is a central area for the reception of all specimens, regardless of their ultimate destination. At St Elsewhere's, with the exception of histopathology samples from the operating theatres, all specimens go to the central pathology reception (Figure 9.4). The contents of the procedure for the central pathology reception [LP-GEN-SpecRec] is shown in Figure 9.14 and covers specimen reception and data acquisition. It also includes the arrangements for subsequent dispatch to the different disciplines/departments within pathology and support for the phlebotomy and courier services.

---

0 INTRODUCTION
    0.1 Purpose and scope
    0.2 Responsibility
    0.3 References
    0.4 Definitions
    0.5 Documentation

1 SPECIMEN RECEPTION
    1.1 Identification of requests and samples
    1.2 Receipt and unpacking of samples from the pneumatic tube
    1.3 Receipt and unpacking of postal samples

2 SPECIMEN REJECTION
    2.1 Criteria for rejection of samples
    2.2 Record of samples rejected and further action taken

3 DATA ACQUISITION
    3.1 Patient identification data
    3.2 Examination request data

4 REFERRAL LABORATORIES
    4.1 Data logging (see section 3)
    4.2 Specimen dispatch [LP-GEN-RefLabs]
    4.3 Receipt of reports

5 STOCK CONTROL AND DISPATCH OF REQUEST FORMS AND SPECIMEN CONTAINERS TO USERS
    5.1 Request forms
    5.2 Specimen containers

6 SUPPORT FOR PHLEBOTOMY/ COURIER SERVICES
    6.1 Production of collection lists from the LIS
    6.2 Cleaning and stocking of phlebotomy trolleys
    6.3 Cleaning of courier transport boxes

Figure 9.14 Contents for a procedure for specimen reception [LP-GEN-SpecRec]

ISO 15189:2002 requires that 'criteria shall be developed and documented for acceptance or rejection of primary samples' and 'if compromised primary samples are accepted, the final report shall indicate the nature of the problem and if applicable, that caution is required when interpreting the result'. Specimens or samples can be compromised by uncertain identity (e.g. a request card received with an inadequately labelled specimen container in the same plastic envelope) or by inadequacy of the specimen (e.g. analysis vitiated by haemolysis). Mechanisms for categorising and recording these incidents will enable corrective and/or preventative action to be taken. It is crucial that clinicians are informed if a specimen is compromised or rejected and reasons for the action taken provided. It is not satisfactory for this notification to be left until a report is issued. The procedure for specimen reception should detail the action to be taken and no specimen should be discarded until the clinician has been informed.

As can be seen from Figure 9.4, the procedure for specimen reception interlocks with the procedure(s) for referring samples to referral laboratories in such a way that samples are dispatched from the central pathology reception, but the reports from the referral laboratories go via central reception to the individual departments before being issued. The Histopathology Department receives specimens by transit through the central pathology reception or directly via the portering service. The reception process being managed by a separate procedure [LP-HIS-SpecRec] specific for Histopathology.

At St Elsewhere's the Pathology Department encourages the request card and specimen container to be closely associated during transportation by providing specially designed polythene bags with separate compartments for specimen container(s) and request form. This is also good health and safety practice. During the process of initial sorting of specimens, care should be taken not to disassociate the relationship between the request form and specimen. Only if unique identification was available for the sample container at the time of collection will the association be absolute. In most laboratories it is the practice to assign a label with an accession number (and sometimes other information, such as patient's name and tests required) to both the request form and the specimen container on arrival. Many laboratory computer systems allow the entry of patient identification data and the tests requested into the computer, which subsequently produces unique labels for the specimen container and request form. The procedure should ensure that such labels do not obscure any information already inscribed on the specimen container label or the request form, so that subsequent checks can be made to confirm the relationship between the request and the specimen.

It is not uncommon to find that the specimen reception and data acquisition functions are undertaken by junior members of the laboratory staff and a large part of the work is extremely repetitive. It is, therefore, important to arrange some variety in the duties of such personnel and to ensure a training programme, that not only teaches the task to be performed, but also emphasises the critical importance of the work being undertaken, and finally to ensure a high level of supervision.

The term data is sometimes used interchangeably with information, but in this section it is used in a more restricted sense as being any series of observations, measurements or facts. This acquisition of data continues throughout the examination process until the reporting and interpretation stage, when it undergoes transformation into information or 'what the data conveys'. This is an important aspect of reporting because until a particular observation or measurement is interpreted, by comparing the observation in the case of histopathology against what is known to occur in a particular pathological condition, or in the case of quantitative measurements referring to appropriate reference intervals, it lacks the value necessary to make it useful in patient care. Accurate acquisition of data and its presentation as information is not only important for this prime purpose of effective patient care, but is also important for a range of management and business purposes, such as how many reagents to purchase for a particular analyzer and in some cases where to send the bill!

If the laboratory is not computerised then it will be necessary to maintain a record book in which details of the specimen(s) received and the identification of the patient are carefully recorded. Such records are often known as day books and are still maintained in some departments in addition to the computer record. With increasing demands upon pathology departments, however, this is only possible in those departments such as histopathology which receive relatively few requests, albeit the requests result in a large amount of work.

REFERRAL TO OTHER LABORATORIES
'Ideal Standard' clause 7.1.6 Referral to other laboratories
Both ISO 17125:1999 clause 4.5, *'Sub-contracting of tests and calibrations'*, and ISO 15189:2002, clause 4.5 *'Examination by referral laboratories'*, invoke the necessity most laboratories have to refer tests or examinations to other laboratories. A 'referral laboratory' is defined in ISO 15189:2002 as an 'external laboratory to which a sample is submitted for a supplementary or confirmatory examination procedure and report'. The sample can be an aliquot of serum, a block of tissue or a stained or unstained section on a slide. The referring laboratory might require a number of different types of service; investigations or tests rarely performed by the referring laboratory, confirmation of initial unusual findings, the provision of a backup service to the referring laboratory in the event of a planned or unforeseen interruption of service, or lastly referral of routine tests as part of a rationalisation of services between two or more laboratories.

A major concern in accreditation standards about referral for specialised investigations is that the work should be undertaken in an approved or controlled facility and the NPAAC Standard 5, 'Pre-analytical phase' draws particular attention to the fact that 'where a sample is referred to another laboratory the specimen must conform to the requirements of the referral laboratory, such as collection procedures, processing of the specimen; and transport conditions'. The key requirements in ISO 15189:2002 in relation to referral to other laboratories are summarised in Figure 9.15.

The referral of **examinations to referral laboratories** requires that...

- the referring laboratory has a procedure for evaluating and selecting referral laboratories, including consultants who are to provide second opinions for histopathology, cytology and related disciplines

- referral arrangements are reviewed periodically and documented

- a register be kept of all referring laboratories and consultants providing second opinions

- a record be kept of samples referred and copy of the record kept in the patient's record and in the referring laboratory

- the referring laboratory be responsible for ensuring the report is returned to the requester and that it contains all essential elements of the results from the referral laboratory, without alterations that could affect clinical interpretation

- interpretative comments may be added by the referring laboratory, but the author of any additional comments should be clearly identified

based upon the ISO 15189:2002 clause 4.5 Examination by referral laboratories

---

Figure 9.15 Requirements for referral laboratories

A further requirement in relation to the reporting of results from referral laboratories appears in ISO 15189:2002 in clause 5.8 *'Reporting of results'* which says 'when examinations from a referral laboratory need to be transcribed by the referring laboratory, procedures to verify the correctness of all transcriptions shall be in place'.

The NCCLS have prepared a guideline on this topic entitled, 'Selecting and Evaluating a Referral Laboratory'. It seeks to identify objective criteria by which a laboratory could be judged. Most of the criteria are similar to those for any laboratory seeking to comply with the standards set by a recognised quality or accreditation system, but included in the checklist is the concept of the referral laboratory's reputation starting with the question 'Will the laboratory provide a list of key clients for you to contact?' One of the most important reasons for the referral of a specimen for a unique or unusual investigation is to benefit from the interpretative and clinical advice available in such centres, e.g. in the case of certain bone tumours, gut hormones or phage typing. Such knowledge is often built from personal contacts and it is not always possible to evaluate this objectively.

EXAMINATION PROCESSES
'Ideal Standard' clause 7.2 Examination processes
see Chapter 10

POST-EXAMINATION PROCESSES
'Ideal Standard' clause 7.3 Post- examination processes
The overall purpose of all post-examination activities is to ensure that the results of examinations are presented accurately and clearly and reach the user in a timely and secure manner. Figure 9.2 indicates that there are clauses of ISO 17025:1999 and ISO 15189:2002, dealing with reporting results, (5.10 and 5.8), in part with validation and authorization (4.9 and 5.7) and with clinical advice and interpretation (4.7). The material will be presented in the following sections in a process related manner.

REPORTING RESULTS
'Ideal Standard' clause 7.3.1 Reporting results
The reporting of results involves three main issues, a) the content and presentation of the report, b) responsibility for its validation and authorization, and c) method and security of communication and ownership.

CONTENT AND PRESENTATION
In ISO 15189:2002 emphasis is placed on the results (reports) being legible, without mistakes in transcription, and that they should be sent to personnel authorized to receive and use medical information. The requirements for report content specified in ISO 15189:2002 are summarised in Figure 9.16 and it is further required that the descriptions of examinations should be in the vocabulary and syntax recommended by professional and other organizations. As has been said in the section on specimen reception and data acquisition, it is how data is presented on the final report that determines its value as information. In disciplines where the results are in the form of observations, bodies such as the College of American Pathologists and the Royal College of Pathologists in the UK recommend standardized procedures (protocols) for reporting the findings of macroscopic and microscopic findings. Information on these protocols and on a similar approach to microbiology reporting by the PHLS is detailed in Appendix 2, Further reading.

The report should ideally include but not be limited to the...

- identification of the laboratory issuing the report (and if different the identity of the laboratory undertaking the investigation)

- report destination

- identification of the requester (and their address)

- identification and location of the patient

- date and time of primary sample collection

- date and time of receipt by the laboratory

- date and time of issuing the report

- type of primary sample and its source

- results of the examination including information on factors (e.g. haemolysis, inadequate labelling of specimen container) that could compromise the results

- biological reference intervals where applicable

- interpretive comments, where appropriate

- indentity of the person authorizing the report

Figure 9.16 The report content

VALIDATION AND AUTHORIZATION

To establish that data and information is correct and appropriate, and to authorize it for release, is an important part of reporting and the processes involved should be defined in a written procedure(s). It is common to talk about two types of validation, often termed technical and clinical validation. The definition of validation provided in Figure 8.9 is 'confirmation by examination and provision of objective evidence that the particular requirements for a specific intended use are fulfilled'. It is not easy to define the difference between technical and clinical validation, but it could be seen as relating to interpretation of the phrase 'specific intended use'. If the specific intended use is seen as 'providing information' to assist in the diagnosis of disease etc. (Figure 9.5), then technical validation relates to confirming that, 'requirements set for the examination in terms of its performance', have been met. These would include the results of calibrations and internal quality control being within pre-specified limits or that observations recorded on tape have been correctly transcribed. Indeed such activities might be best regarded as part of the examination rather than the post-examination process.

If, however, the specific intended use is seen as 'fulfilling the reason for ordering of the test' e.g. the diagnosis of disease, then the term clinical validation is perhaps more appropriate as it implies bringing together the results of the examination and the clinical information available and validating that the 'reason for ordering the test' has been fulfilled. This clinical or medical validation, often called 'signing out' of reports, is performed by a senior member of the medical or scientific staff.

Some technical validation can be done automatically and only nonconformities drawn to the attention of the technical verifier. For example, a report dependent on observations, such as the macroscopic and microscopic descriptions of tissue submitted for analysis, can be checked using a spell checker or, going back one stage, the report can in part be produced by automatic incorporation of phrases using brief mnemonics, such as 'spcon' equals 'The specimen consists of....'. The provision or ability to create a specialised or personal dictionary, against which the spell checking is done, is a normal part of present day computer systems.

Quantitative measurements can be subjected to checks which can activate different responses. If a haemoglobin or serum potassium result is outside one set of limits it can be flagged prior to reporting, as incompatible with life, or in other words a 'nonsense report'. These technical checks can be done without a computerised system but, as the volume of data produced per week by even a small laboratory is large, there are clearly limitations on what can be achieved.

Some methods, normally considered as technical validation, such as a result being in a critical area, can be used to select particular results for the further process of clinical validation. The validation by scrutiny of a group of results for internal consistency can be achieved using rule-based algorithms which can decide that 'normally' a high result for one examination is incompatible with a low result for a second examination, and flag that situation for attention. Logically the final clinical validation, albeit retrospective, is the involvement of the laboratory in clinical audit and effectiveness studies (see Chapter 11).

COMMUNICATION OF REPORTS

Reports can be communicated either by hard copy or electronically, but each method has its particular problems in terms of the content remaining uncorrupted (fidelity) and it being securely transferred (security). Fidelity is usefully defined in this context in electronic terms, as 'the extent to which the output signal accurately reproduces the characteristics of the input signal'. Paper copy reports are unlikely to have their content corrupted during dispatch, but the mechanism by which they reach the patient's record needs to be clearly defined. St Elsewhere's undertakes a regular audit of the speed of delivery of postal and courier services, of reports sent to out-patients and wards and their safe arrival in the patient's record.

The important NPAAC publication, 'Guidelines for data communication', contains much straightforward and practical advice on a subject of emerging complexity and importance. It deals with the key issues of the principles of privacy, fidelity and security of communication, the definition of responsibilities and boundaries, inter-operability *(technical standards)*, and audit trails. Guideline 2, 'Fidelity and security of information' defines four methods of electronic pathology communications: laboratory initiated or requester initiated message communication *(the telephoned report)*, file transfer by physical media, direct access by outside to the pathology system, and faxing (manual or automatic).

The guideline further comments in relation to these methods that, 'unauthorized physical or electronic access and sending information to the wrong destination would appear to have the highest risk'. However, the 'telephoned report' presents particular risks in terms of both fidelity and security as any reader who has participated in the party game of 'passing the message' will understand. ISO 15189:2002 requires in clause 5.8 that 'the laboratory shall establish policies and practices to ensure that results distributed by telephone or other electronic means only reach an authorized receiver' and goes on to stipulate that 'results provided verbally shall be followed by a properly recorded report'. At St Elsewhere's, the procedure for reporting results [LP-GEN-Reports] includes a section on 'the telephoned report' based upon requirements specified in CPA Standard G3 (Figure 9.17). This aims to minimise the risks associated with verbal communication and establishes an audit trail should investigation of errors be required.

OWNERSHIP AND PRIVACY

Pathology organizations throughout the world are taking an increasingly stringent approach to the protection of patient information. In the United Kingdom this is based upon the recommendations of the Caldicott Committee, 'Report on the review of patient-identifiable information', the General Medical Council (GMC) publication, 'Confidentiality: Protecting and Providing Information' and upon the recent guidance on the application of the Data Protection Act 1998 on the 'Use and Disclosure of Health Data'. The DoH in UK have produced a 'Manual for Caldicott Guardians' which summarises the six principles of the Caldicott Report with regard to the patient-identifiable information that are set out in Figure 9.18.

G3 The telephoned report

Laboratories are frequently required to telephone reports to users. The method by which this is done needs to be clearly defined to minimise the risk of error.

G 3.1   Laboratory management shall establish a procedure(s) for giving reports by telephone which includes:

a) the circumstances in which reports may be given
b) the nominated individuals who may give reports
c) the individuals who may receive reports
d) a method of mutual identification of the patient between reporter and receiver
e) a confirmation of correct transmission
f) the mechanism for recording the event
g) the maintenance of confidentiality
h) the process for sending a follow up report

CPA(UK)Ltd Standards for the Medical Laboratory 2001

Figure 9.17 CPA(UK)Ltd, Standard G3, The telephoned report

Another important issue related to ownership is dealt with in the RCPath publication on 'advice relating to the ownership, storage and release of pathology results'. It includes advice on the release of results directly to patients and to doctor-patients. This is in the form of a commentary on the potential problems of giving out individual pathology results to individual patients (Figure 9.19).

At St Elsewhere's, the Pathology Laboratory is grappling with the implementation of these recommendations and has set up a training programme to enable staff to understand the implications for pathology. At present results are only given to the requestor and doctors are not allowed to request examinations on themselves. No direct access to the laboratory information system is allowed by users of the Pathology Laboratory, and all electronic messaging and file transfer of patient's reports being done via the hospital order communications system, is subject to scrutiny by the Caldicott Guardian. At St Elsewhere's, the Medical Director of the hospital, who undertakes this role, is a member of the Trust Management Board and responsible for clinical governance.

- **Principle 1 - Justify the purpose(s)**

  Every proposed use or transfer of patient-identifiable information within or from an organization should be clearly defined and scrutinised, with continuing uses regularly reviewed by an appropriate guardian.

- **Principle 2 - Don't use patient-identifiable information unless it is absolutely necessary**

  Patient-identifiable information items should not be used unless there is no alternative.

- **Principle 3 - Use the minimum necessary patient-identifiable information**

  Where use of patient-identifiable information items is considered to be essential, each individual item of information should be justified with the aim of reducing identifiability.

- **Principle 4 - Access to patient-identifiable information should be on a strict need to know basis**

  Only those individuals who need access to patient-identifiable information should have access to it, and they should only have access to the information items they need to see.

- **Principle 5 - Everyone should be aware of their responsibilities**

  Action should be taken to ensure that those handling patient-identifiable information - both clinical and non-clinical staff - are aware of their responsibilities and obligations to observe patient confidentiality.

- **Principle 6 - Understand and comply with the law**

  Every use of patient-identifiable information must be lawful. Someone in each organization should be responsible for ensuring that the organization complies with legal requirements.

Figure 9.18 The Caldicott principles

Potential problems related to giving out **individual pathology results directly to patients,** include...

a) the difficulty of establishing that they are who they say they are and hence ensuring confidentiality

b) the problem of giving individual results in isolation to someone who might not understand their nature or misinterpret their significance

c) particular sensitivities over certain results, such as HIV tests or biopsies for suspected malignancy, which have serious clinical significance

d) the possibility of undermining the established relationship between the patient and clinician primarily responsible for their care

based on 'Advice relating to the ownership, storage and release of pathology results'
Royal College of Pathologists UK 2001

Figure 9.19 Release of pathology results to patients

CLINICAL ADVICE AND INTERPRETATION
'Ideal Standard' clause 7.3.2 Clinical advice and interpretation
In ISO 15189:2002, clause 4.7 says that 'appropriate laboratory professional staff shall provide advice on choice of examinations and use of the services, including repeat frequency and required type of sample. Where appropriate, interpretation of the results of examinations shall be provided'. Standard 2 of the NPAAC 'Draft Standards for Pathology Laboratories', states the requirement more precisely when it says 'pathologists and other senior staff with appropriate training must be available to provide advice on...' and goes on to give a clear indication of the requirement for the consultative aspect of a laboratory's work, and in particular the evaluation and interpretation of results (Figure 9.20).

In some disciplines, such as histopathology, the interpretative comments based on observations are the basis of the report, but in other disciplines it is important to undertake an objective assessment of their value and, in particular, their effect on the action taken by the clinician receiving the comments. A comment which might be helpful to a primary care clinician regarding the significance of a thyroid function test might be seen as irrelevant or even insulting to an endocrinologist. Comments which warn the clinician that something was amiss in the collection of the sample, i.e. haemolysis or incomplete labelling of the sample are an obligatory feature of good reporting. External quality assessment schemes that assess interpretative comments will be discussed in Chapter 11.

STANDARD 2 - STAFFING, SUPERVISION AND **CONSULTATION**

There shall be staff who can advise on the selection of tests, the evaluation and interpretation of laboratory results and the validity of the methods employed in the laboratory.

COMMENTARY

- Pathologists and other senior staff with appropriate training and experience must be available to provide advice on:
  - the clinical significance of results,
  - the interpretation and correlation of laboratory data,
  - the suitability of tests and procedures in various clinical situations, and
  - appropriate further tests and procedures

selected from Standard 2, Draft Standards for Pathology Laboratories, NPAAC (2001)

Figure 9.20   NPAAC Standard 2 – Staffing, supervision and consultation

CONTROL OF CLINICAL MATERIAL
'Ideal Standard' clause 4.2.5 Control of clinical material

GENERAL

Discussion of this topic has been postponed from Chapter 5 as it seems to fit more logically in a discussion of post-examination process. However, it still remains an important part of a quality management system, with the same significance as clause 4.2.4 of the 'Ideal Standard' on controlling records. Indeed artifacts created during the examination process, such as slides and blocks and electrophoretic gels, can be considered as *records* of an examination process. The use of the term 'clinical material' in this text is intended to include both human organs and human tissue. In the 'Good practice in consent implementation guide' published by the DoH UK, the term human tissue is taken to include 'blood samples and other bodily fluids provided for testing'.

The primary reason for having a system for the control of clinical material is to make it possible to reconstruct an examination process, either by re-examining existing artifacts or recreating the examination process itself.

The contents of a procedure for control of clinical material is shown in Figure 9.21 and seeks to fulfil the requirements described. Many of the considerations governing the control of clinical material are the same as those governing the control of (patient) records and the following discussion highlights some of the specific issues dealt with by the procedure. Because of the sensitive public issues concerning this procedure, the Pathology Management Board of St Elsewhere's require the overall responsibility for this procedure to be with the Director of Pathology in conjunction with the heads of departments.

---

0   INTRODUCTION
   0.1   Purpose and scope
   0.2   Responsibility
   0.3   References
   0.4   Definitions
   0.5   Documentation

1   CONSENT
   1.1   Requirements of the laboratory
   1.2   Requirements of St Elsewhere's Hospital Trust
   1.3   Requirements of legislation
   1.4   Information for patients [PD-MOR-InfoPMs] and [PD-GEN-SpecCol]

2   TYPE OF CLINICAL MATERIAL AND RETENTION TIMES [MF-GEN-ClinMat]
   2.1   Haematology
   2.2   Biochemistry
   2.3   Microbiology
   2.4   Histopathology
   2.5   Cytology

3   REGISTRATION, IDENTIFICATION AND INDEXING
   3.1   Registration
   3.2   Identification
   3.3   Indexing

4   CONFIDENTIALITY AND SECURITY
   4.1   Conditions for alternative uses
   4.2   Confidentiality
   4.3   Security arrangements

5   STORAGE AND RETRIEVAL
   5.1   On-site
   5.2   Off-site

6   RELEASE AND DISPOSAL
   6.1   Release to relatives
   6.2   Release to third parties
   6.3   On-site
   6.4   External contractors

7   AUDIT OF CONTROL OF CLINICAL MATERIAL

Figure 9.21 Contents of a procedure for control of clinical material [MP-GEN-MatCtrl]

CONSENT
Any procedure for control and retention of clinical material needs to refer to, or have within it, information concerning patient consent. The current advice for hospital trusts in the UK follows the spirit of the Articles detailed in Figure 9.7 and 'requires that patients be given the right to refuse permission for tissue taken from them at surgery or other procedure to be used for education or research purposes', but in relation to tissue samples used for quality assurance (including blood) suggests that specific patient consent need not be sought, *'providing* there

is an active policy of informing patients of such use'. At St Elsewhere's patients attention is drawn to a notice (Figure 9.22), displayed in all areas where phlebotomy takes place.

PATHOLOGY LABORATORY, ST ELSEWHERE'S HOSPITAL TRUST

**IMPORTANT NOTICE TO ALL PATIENTS HAVING
BLOOD SAMPLES TAKEN FOR LABORATORY EXAMINATION**

Your doctor has requested a blood test. The blood collector will take no more blood than we think will be necessary to complete all the procedures which have been requested. However, in many cases a small amount of blood is left over when we have completed our tests.

This surplus blood is vital material for laboratories. We use it for teaching purposes, to check the quality of our laboratory systems, to determine the normal levels of blood constituents and in research projects. All our research projects are strictly regulated by the Trust's ethical committee, which looks after the interests of individual patients.

We very much hope that you will have no objection to use of surplus material in this way, and will assume this is the case for all samples received in the normal manner. However, if you do have any objection to the use of surplus material, please ask the blood collector to record your objection on the request form, and we will ensure that your wishes are respected.

Thank you very much for your help. If you would like any further information, please contact:

Dr William Jaggard,
Director of Pathology,
St Elsewhere's Hospital Trust,
Eastside Street,
St ELSEWHERE
East Loanshire EL7 5XX

PD-GEN-SpecCol January 2002

Figure 9.22 Consent for phlebotomy – alternative uses

This notice is registered in Q-Pulse as public document [PD-GEN-SpecCol], as is the information for relatives concerning post-mortems [PD-MOR-InfoPMs] (Figure 9.8).

CLINICAL MATERIAL AND RETENTION TIMES

Decisions regarding the retention of clinical material are made by the heads of individual departments, but because of the difficulties encountered in the past by St Elsewhere's Hospital Trust, the Pathology Management Board formally agrees the decisions, which are based on the best current advice available. In order that the situation can be easily reviewed, records of type of specimen, retention time and long term storage arrangements specific to each department, are kept on a form [MF-GEN-ClinMat], an example of which is shown in Figure 9.23. These records are reviewed every twelve months and revised as necessary.

RETENTION OF CLINICAL MATERIAL FORM

RECORD FILENAME	MF-HAE-ClinMat#Haematology

1 Department	2 Section
Haematology	Routine

3 Head of Department	4 Section supervisor
Dr Theresa Hone	Bob Long

5 Records

Type of clinical material	Retention time	Storage conditions	Location	Indexing
All specimens unless specifically mentioned below	7 days from date of receipt or until 2 days after the date of the issued report	Refrigerated 4°C	Routine refrigerator (labelled SPECIMEN S1)	by day of receipt
Reported blood film	As above if film NORMAL If film findings SIGNIFICANT, 1 year	Room temperature, 18°C	Slide cabinet in laboratory (labelled FILMS F1)	by accession number
Routine blood samples	2 days	Room temperature, 18°C	Routine laboratory	by day of receipt
Bone marrow slides	2 years	Room temperature, 18°C	Slide cabinet in laboratory (labelled MARROW C1)	by accession number

Figure 9.23 Retention of clinical material form [MF-GEN-ClinMat]

The NPAAC and the RCPath have produced guidelines for the retention of clinical material which contain much useful information and it is an informative exercise to compare the recommendations before deciding on retention times. It is important that decisions taken regarding retention are in accordance with local requirements and in compliance with national legislation and regulations.

REGISTRATION, IDENTIFICATION AND INDEXING
Identification and indexing is important for the speedy and efficient retrieval of specimens and artifacts for internal purposes of re-examination. However, in relation to retention of clinical material from post-mortem examinations a more detailed record needs to be kept that includes, in addition to the usual information about the specimen, the ability to record, with signatures, the date of release to a *bone fide* relative or friend.

CONFIDENTIALITY AND SECURITY
If specimens are to be released to a third party for research or quality assurance purposes then they need to be de-identified in order that they cannot be traced back to the patient. This equally applies to any records accompanying them.

RELEASE AND DISPOSAL
The release of material retained from post-mortems to a *bone fide* relative or friend needs to be handled with sensitivity. At St Elsewhere's, section 6.1 'Release to relatives' is written to comply with the advice from the NPAAC (Figure 4.3) that the laboratory should 'have policies and procedures to ensure there are acceptable standards of staff conduct towards human samples, tissues or remains'. All destructive disposal should be secure and in compliance with the host organization's waste disposal procedures.

Chapter 10

Examination process

INTRODUCTION
'Ideal Standard' clause 7.2 Examination process
In the introduction to Chapter 9 it was stressed that the examination processes include pre- and post-examination processes. In this chapter the focus is on the examination or analytical process and includes a brief section on point-of-care testing (POCT). Figure 9.2 showed the clauses of ISO 15189:2002 and ISO 17025:1999 that relate to the examination process. The comparable clause in ISO 9001:2000, is 7.5 *'Production and service provision'*. Figure 10.1 shows the inter-relationships between the 'examination process' clauses of the 'Ideal Standard' and clauses from the 'evaluation and improvement' section of the standard that relate to assurance. It can be seen from the diagram that there are three distinct aspects to the examination process; the selection and validation of procedures, the procedures themselves and assuring the quality of results that are produced by the use of these procedures.

SELECTION AND VALIDATION
'Ideal Standard' clause 7.2.1 Selection and validation
The questions involved in the selection and validation of examination procedures are closely inter-related. In Chapter 8 the process of IVD procurement was discussed. What follows on selection and validation of examination procedures is an extension of that discussion, and applies equally to the periodic re-evaluation/re-validation of examination procedures already in use in the laboratory.

There are three questions to be asked: 'What is the intended clinical use of the proposed new examination?' (see Figure 9.5), 'will the examination fulfil its intended clinical use?' and, 'will the (technical) performance of the examination provide the information required to fulfil its intended use?'. The second and third questions involve a process of validation akin to the concept of clinical and technical validation discussed under post-examination processes in Chapter 9.

It is important to determine the extent to which the medical laboratory (providing a routine service) should and can be involved in these questions, both in terms of complying with international standards and as part of the process of managing quality. In relation to the first question, 'what is the intended clinical use of the proposed new examination?'; the laboratory has to be engaged with clinical staff in determining the intended clinical use of a proposed new examination. To establish a new method for measuring Myocard Z without knowing its intended use, would be untenable. Such information should form part of the assessment of the need for any new IVD (see Figure 8.6).

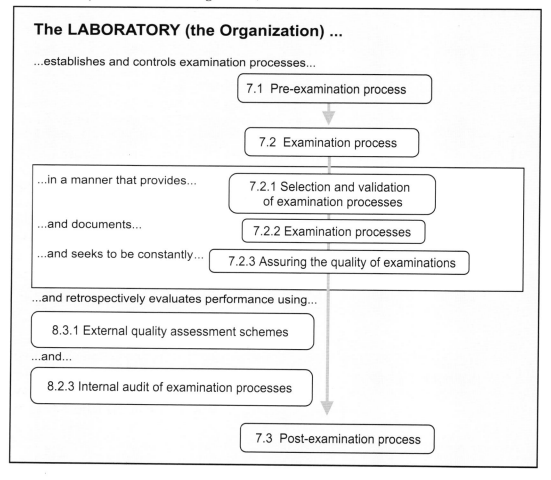

Figure 10.1 Clause 7.2 of the 'Ideal Standard' – Examination process

WILL THE EXAMINATION FULFIL ITS INTENDED CLINICAL USE?/CLINICAL VALIDATION

It is beyond the resources of any one routine medical laboratory to answer the question 'will the examination fulfil its intended clinical use?' and therefore provide a 'clinical validation'. However, it is important that a laboratory provides evidence, through its continuing medical education programme (e.g. attendance at appropriate meetings, conferences and exhibitions), that the selection and re-evaluation of examination procedures takes place in relation to current knowledge.

The Histopathology department at St Elsewhere's has recently drawn the attention of the Pathology Laboratory to a report from the RCPath UK, Histopathology Working Group entitled 'Histopathology of limited or no clinical value'. The remit was to 'initiate a series of evidence-based multidisciplinary evaluations of investigations of doubtful clinical utility to identify those that make little or no contribution to patient care and welfare' and comments further that 'some diagnoses made traditionally by histology may be made with higher sensitivity and specificity by other methods, thus relieving histopathologists of some of their burden'. The recommendations of this report have been adopted by the Pathology Management Board and the application of this approach to the rest of pathology is part of the on-going agenda for the laboratory's management review, (see Chapter 11).

An important review in the Bandolier, entitled 'Evidence and diagnostics' not only provides valuable key references, but an important analysis of the crucial issues involved in trying to answer the question 'Will the examination fulfil its intended clinical use?'. In the final paragraph headed, 'Where do we go from here?' it states 'If you are in a hole, stop digging. What we are doing now is so awful that we have to scrap most of it and start afresh. Doing systematic reviews is a complete waste of time'. After making some suggestions which are summarised in Figure 10.2, it puts forward a challenge that refreshingly includes the possibility of St Elsewhere's being a part of the process, 'One thing is certain. This should be one of the most fertile areas for research in the next few years. Laboratory scientists, clinicians, nurses, pharmacists and others all should be able to take part. It doesn't need a brain the size of the planet. It doesn't have to be done in some ivory tower, and much could be done in Grimsby on a wet Tuesday afternoon. Watch this space'. The response from Grimsby is not noted, but at St Elsewhere's we are watching this space!

WILL THE PERFORMANCE OF THE EXAMINATION PROCEDURE PROVIDE THE INFORMATION REQUIRED TO FULFIL ITS INTENDED USE?/TECHNICAL VALIDATION

The main concern of ISO 17025:1999 and ISO 15189:2002 in clause 5.4 *'Test and calibration methods and method validation'* and 5.5 *'Examination procedures'* respectively, is with technical validation. In order to conduct a technical validation two issues have to be considered. Firstly, the requirements for performance of an examination have to be established, 'What are the performance requirements that need to be validated?'. Secondly, to what extent should the medical laboratory be involved in these time consuming processes in order to comply with international standards, 'What should be validated and who should undertake the validation?'. EURACHEM, an organization that provides a 'focus for analytical chemistry in Europe', has published a comprehensive laboratory guide to method validation and related topics entitled 'The Fitness for Purpose of Analytical Methods'. This guide interprets the ISO definition of validation for 'method validation', as being 'the process of defining the analytical requirement and confirming that the method under consideration has the performance capabilities consistent with what the application requires'.

- If we do new studies, they must be free from bias. Consecutive patients in real situations is the only way to test tests.

- Studies have to be large to avoid random error.

- Use the Internet, like CARE (www.carestudy.com) to recruit many centres and do things faster.

- Combine clinical and laboratory findings.

- Choose clinical situations where doctors need most help.

- Find better ways of giving results, not normal ranges but algorithms. Start work on new ways of expressing outcomes of diagnostic tests.

- Make results available through better communication.

based on Evidence and diagnostics, Bandolier Extra 2002 (www.ebandolier.com)

Figure 10.2 Evidence and diagnostics – where do we go from here?

Most of what is described in the following sections appears only to apply to quantitative examination procedures, but the same principles apply equally to pre-examination processes involving specimen collection (sampling), transportation, handling and reception of the specimens (integrity and identification) and to examination procedures based on observations. The European Co-operation for Accreditation are currently revising a guide on 'Accreditation for Microbiological Laboratories' that interprets the requirements of ISO 17025:1999 for the discipline of microbiology (see Appendix 2 Further reading). Among much useful advice is specific advice concerning validation, 'Qualitative microbiological test methods, such as where the result is expressed in terms of detected/not detected, and confirmation and identification procedures should be validated by determining, if appropriate, the specificity, relative trueness, positive deviation, negative deviation, limit of deviation, limit of detection, matrix effects, repeatability and reproducibility'. The less well known of these concepts, are carefully defined in an appendix of the publication.

It is also important that the validation of examination procedures, including sampling etc. should not be regarded as a 'once only' activity. In Chapter 8, in the section on validation of computers, it was said that validation should not be regarded as a static phenomenon but rather as an ongoing exercise associated with controlling change (change control). This will be discussed further in the section on 'Assuring the quality of examinations'.

WHAT ARE THE PERFORMANCE REQUIREMENTS THAT NEED TO BE VALIDATED?
The determination of performance goals for examination processes, particularly in relation to quantitative measurements, has been the subject of extensive debate culminating in the Stockholm Consensus Conference on 'Quality Specifications in Laboratory Medicine', 25-26 April 1999 (see Appendix 2 Further reading). An ISO Technical Report (ISO 151960), entitled 'Determination of analytical performance goals for laboratory procedures based upon medical requirements', is in preparation. The need for such performance goals has been set out as shown in Figure 10.3.

The need for **analytical goals of performance** relates to...

- laboratories drawing up specifications or tender documents for new analytical methodology or equipment

- the performance of evaluation studies, to compare values found to those desired

- plan, establish and use quality control programmes in individual laboratories

- help the organizers of external quality assessment schemes design and execute appropriate programmes

- assist manufacturers of instruments and reagents in design, construction and marketing

- and most important of all, to ensure that the analytical quality attained is such that adequate patient care is provided

based on Introduction; Strategies to set global specifications in laboratory medicine
Scand J Clin Lab Invest 1999; 59: 477

Figure 10.3 The need for analytical goals of performance

Although the main focus in this chapter will be on the management of analytical quality, any system of quality performance standards has to include requirements for clinical outcome criteria and analytical outcome criteria in addition to analytical performance criteria. For practical applications these need to be translated into 'operating specifications for the imprecision, inaccuracy, control rules and number of control measurements that are necessary to assure *(ensure)* analytical quality during the routine production of test results'.

The Consensus statement from the Stockholm Conference sets out a hierachy of models that should be applied to set analytical quality specifications. These models are summarised in Figure 10.4. Models higher up the hierarchy being preferred to those lower down.

---

1. Evaluation of the effect of analytical performance on clinical outcomes in a specific clinical setting

2. Evaluation of the effect of analytical performance on clinical decisions in general:
   a. Data based on the components of biological variation
   b. Data based on the analysis of clinicians opinions

3. Published professional recommendations
   a. From national and international expert groups
   b. From expert local groups or individuals

4. Performance goals set by
   a. Regulatory bodies
   b. Organizers of External Quality Assessment (EQA) schemes

5. Goals based on the current state of the art
   a. As demonstrated by data from EQA or Proficiency testing schemes
   b. Organizers of External Quality Assessment (EQA) schemes

   based on Kenny D *et al* Consensus agreement Scand J Clin Lab Invest 1999; 59: 585

Figure 10.4 Hierarchy of models to be applied to set analytical quality specifications

WHAT SHOULD BE VALIDATED AND WHO SHOULD UNDERTAKE THE VALIDATION?
ISO 17025:1999 distinguishes three types of methods, a) methods published in international, regional or national standards and states that these 'shall be preferably used' (referred to as 'standard methods' in this text), b) laboratory developed methods and c) non-standard methods. It expands the definition of 'standard methods', saying that when the client (user) does not specify the method to be used, (largely the case in medical laboratories) that 'the laboratory shall select appropriate methods that have been published either in international, regional or national standards, or by reputable professional organizations, or relevant scientific texts or journals, or as specified by the manufacturer of the equipment'. ISO 15189:2002 states that 'preferred procedures are those that have been published in established/authoritative textbooks, peer reviewed texts or journals, or as international, national or regional guidelines'.

In relation to laboratory developed methods and non-standard methods, there is clear requirement for validation before use and full documentation. However in relation to 'standard methods', ISO 17025:1999 states that 'the laboratory should confirm that it can properly operate standard methods before introducing tests or calibrations'. ISO 15189:2002, with less clarity, requires that 'the laboratory shall only use validated procedures to confirm that the examination procedures are suitable for use', but leaves some room for interpretation when it says ' the validations should be as extensive as are necessary to meet the needs in the given application or field of application'. It is clear that whatever type of level of validation is performed, it must be properly documented and recorded.

With the advent of the IVD Directive and its requirements (Figure 8.3) upon manufacturers to produce data to demonstrate performance claims in relation to certain criteria and the conformity assessment routes for CE marking, full validation in the laboratory would seem not only impracticable, but also unnecessary. The concept in ISO 17025:1999 of confirming 'that it can properly operate standard methods' would seem more realistic. As it is clear that manufacturer's methods can be regarded as 'standard methods', major effort should be put into the selection and procurement processes described in Chapter 8 in order to establish the 'validated status' of the IVD prior to purchase.

A number of European Standards have been produced in response to the requirements of the IVD Directive. The scope of EN 13612:2002 'Performance evaluation of in vitro diagnostic medical devices', states that 'it specifies the responsibilities and general requirements for the planning, conduct, assessment and documentation of a performance evaluation study by the manufacturer'. The section on experimental design details special considerations for performance evaluation studies of reagent kits, and these include the techniques detailed in a note to clause 5.4.5 *'Validation of methods'* of ISO 17025:1999 (Figure 10.5), but are broader in approach.

Techniques used to determine the performance of a method should include...

- calibration using reference standards or reference materials

- comparison of results achieved with other methods

- inter-laboratory comparisons

- systematic assessment of the factors influencing the result

- assessment of the uncertainty of the results based on a scientific under-standing of the theoretical principles of the method and practical experience

based on ISO 17025:1999 General requirements for the competence of testing and calibration laboratories

---

Figure 10.5 Techniques to be used to determine performance of a method

The extensive bibliography of EN 13612:2002 provides a valuable resource for specific evaluation plan standards produced by NCCLS (National Committee for Clinical Laboratory Standards, USA), the now defunct ECCLS (European Committee for Clinical Laboratory Standards) and other published works, a selection of which are included in Appendix 2, Further reading. Other related published Standards or Standards in preparation are ISO/DIS 15198 'Clinical laboratory medicine – IVDs – Validation of manufacturer's recommendations for user quality control'; EN 12322:1999 'IVDs – Culture media for microbiology – Performance criteria for culture media' and EN 13640:2002 'Stability testing of in vitro diagnostic reagents'.

EXAMINATION PROCEDURES
'Ideal Standard' clause 7.2.2 Examination procedures

INTRODUCTION
Later in the chapter a practical approach to the preparation of examination procedures will be discussed, but first the requirements of International Standards in relation to examination procedures need to be checked in order to ensure that, whatever approach to the preparation of examination procedures is adopted, the requirements are met. Special issues such as the relationship between preparation for examination and examination itself, risk assessment of examination procedures and uncertainty are discussed, primarily to introduce the concepts and useful references.

ISO 15189:2002 clause 5.5 *'Examination procedures'*, starts by acknowledging that some of the sub-clauses of the section may not apply to all disciplines of laboratory practice. This says in effect, that not all the requirements for examinations involving measurement can be requirements for examinations dependent on observation. However, some requirements are common to all examinations, whether based on measurement or observation. It requires that 'all procedures shall be documented and be available at the workstation for relevant staff' and that all documentation 'shall be available in a language commonly understood by the staff in the laboratory'. It is not unduly prescriptive about the source of the material or how it is presented, but requires that all documentation is part of a document control system and that it should include the items shown in Figure 10.6 (with appropriate exceptions for examinations based on observation).

In the preparation of in-house documentation concerning examinations, or in evaluating any documentation provided by manufacturers, the completeness of any approach should be confirmed by reference to the content of examination documentation shown in Figure 10.6, plus the information required in 'a manufacturer's instructions for use' based on EN 591:2001 (Figure 8.7) and the 'information supplied by manufacturers with in vitro diagnostic reagents' based on EN 375:2001 and shown in Figure 10.7.

Most of the content of EN 375:2001 (Figure 10.7) is self explanatory and cross references to the IVD Directive are given in an appendix. From the point of view of accreditation it is important; a) that in clause 5.14 *'Changes in the procedure and in performance'*, a requirement is placed on the manufacturer to ensure 'that the user is informed of any substantial changes in the procedure and/or analytical performance of the IVD reagent and of measures to be taken in this event', and b) that in clause 5.19 *'Date of issue or revision'*, that 'the date of issue or latest revision of the instructions for use shall be given'. In this connection it is vital the user laboratory keeps the manufacturer or supplier informed of the best way in which to communicate these issues.

a) purpose of the examination
b) principle of the procedure used for examinations
c) performance specifications (e.g. linearity, precision, accuracy expressed as standard uncertainty of measurement, detection limit, measuring interval, trueness expressed as systematic error, analytical sensitivity and analytical specificity)
d) primary sample type (including container and additives)
e) required equipment and reagents; or examining system
f) calibration procedures
g) procedural steps
h) quality control procedures
i) interferences (e.g. lipaemia, haemolysis, bilirubin and cross reactions)
j) principle of procedure for calculating results
k) biological reference intervals
l) reportable interval of patient examination results
m) alert/critical values, where appropriate
n) laboratory interpretation
o) safety precautions
p) potential sources of variability

based on ISO 15189:2002 Medical laboratories – Particular requirements for quality and competence

Clause 5.5 Examination procedures

Figure 10.6 ISO 15189:2002 Content of examination documentation

PREPARATION FOR EXAMINATION AND EXAMINATION

In each department of a pathology laboratory there will be differences in the processes for the preparation of specimens for examination and the examination itself. In histopathology and cytopathology it is difficult to know whether specimen preparation should be regarded as being separate from the examination. Certainly the guidelines used in histopathology for 'cut-up' or 'gross examination' of specimens prior to embedding are a key part of the examination process and contribute to the final report in terms of the macroscopic appearance. Similarly, the preparation of blood films in Haematology and their subsequent fixation and staining is also a major part of the examination process.

5.1	General	5.12	Methodology
5.2	Manufacturer (name and address)		5.12.1 Principle of the method
5.3	Product name		5.12.2 Performance characteristics
5.4	Microbiological state		and limitations of the method
5.5	Intended purpose		5.12.3 Reagent preparation
5.6	Warning and precautions	5.13	Calculation of analytical results
5.7	Composition	5.14	Changes in the procedure and in
5.8	Storage and shelf life after first		the performance
	opening	5.15	Internal quality control
5.9	Additional special equipment	5.16	Traceability of calibrators and
5.10	Specimen		control materials
5.11	Procedure	5.17	Reference intervals
		5.18	Literature references
		5.19	Date of issue or revision

based upon EN 375:2001 'Information supplied by the manufacturer with in vitro diagnostic reagents for professional use' Clause 5 Requirements for instructions for use

Figure 10.7 Requirements for 'information supplied by manufacturers with in vitro diagnostic reagents'

In haematology and biochemistry a specimen/sample is collected for a specific purpose and it is easy to relate that sample to the original request form by giving the sample and the request form a unique accession number. Only occasionally are follow up tests required. Problems in the identification chain can arise when aliquots of the original sample have to be taken because the analyses required are done on two different analyzers. One aliquot might go on an analyzer which reads a bar coded label, and another onto an analyzer where its identity is preserved by relating its order on a work sheet to its position on an instrument carousel. Recent innovations in instrumentation allow aliquoting of the primary sample and assignment of identity automatically. For many analyzers the primary collection container (often an evacuated tube in which the blood sample is collected) can, after centrifugation to separate the serum from the cellular components, be put directly onto the analytical instrument. Whenever this procedure is possible it should be encouraged, as it reduces the opportunity for error that can occur when aliquots of the original sample have to be put into secondary containers prior to analysis.

However, in microbiology and histopathology it is not always clear until after the initial investigation what subsequent investigations will be required, for example, when a urine is submitted for culture or a specimen is sent for histological examination. It is very important to develop a system in which any subsequent investigations can be related to the original specimen presented for examination. For example, a urine might be cultured and three distinct colonies of microorganism require further investigation for identification and also for sensitivity testing. A similar situation occurs in histopathology when one or more biopsy specimens are submitted for investigation and two 'blocks of tissue' are prepared from Specimen 1 and placed in separate cassettes for embedding as paraffin blocks, then paraffin block A is sectioned at two levels to produce sections which are mounted on two slides. It is important to distinguish 'blocks of tissue' from 'paraffin blocks' because Specimen 2 might produce more than one block of tissue, all mounted in one paraffin block.

RISK ASSESSMENT OF EXAMINATION PROCEDURES

In Chapter 7, the identification of hazards in the laboratory and assessment of the potential risks associated with the hazards was discussed (Figure 7.19). The general approach described is equally applicable to examination procedures. However, in relation to examination procedures the particular focus is on the potential risks associated with the biological and chemical agents used in examination procedures. In Europe, Directive 98/24/EC on the protection of the health and safety of workers from the risks related to chemical agents at work, required implementation by Members States of the EU and will lead to a revision, in 2002, of the UK Control of Substances Hazardous to Health (COSHH) Regulations 1999. Similar regulations exist, to greater or lesser extent in content and application, in countries throughout the world. In most countries therefore, the requirement for risk assessment of examination procedures stems, not from the need to comply with standards used by accreditation bodies, but the need to comply with the law of the land. In Section II of the Directive, Article 4 details the obligations of the employer to make a 'Determination and assessment of the risk of hazardous chemical agents' taking into consideration the items shown in Figure 10.8.

At first the work involved seems overwhelming, and it is important to determine a practical approach in order to keep a sense of perspective. Adoption of the 'standard precautions' described in Chapter 7 goes a long way to protect laboratory workers from occupationally acquired infections associated with specimens entering the laboratory. In laboratory practice, potential exposure of laboratory personnel to high levels of chemical agents is limited to the preparatory stages of a process such as weighing or dispensing and not to their routine use. However, the creation of dust or aerosols and mechanisms of waste disposal present further potential risks. It is important to understand the nature of the hazard, for example the risk associated with the ingestion of the radio-isotope tri-iodothyronine might be greater because of its biological activity than because of its radioactivity.

The requirement on the laboratory raises two practical questions. Firstly; 'How should the hazards be evaluated, and risk assessed and recorded? and secondly, 'What to do with the information from the risk assessment?' in order that laboratory workers are aware of the risks and can take appropriate measures to minimise the risk to themselves and others.

...the employer shall first determine whether any hazardous chemical agents are present at the workplace. If so, he shall assess any risk to the health and safety of the workers arising from the presence of those chemical agents, taking into consideration the following:

- their hazardous properties

- information on health and safety that shall be provided by the supplier

- the level, type and duration of exposure

- the circumstances of work involving such agents including their amount

- any occupational exposure limit values or biological limit values established on the territory of the Member State in question

- the effect of preventative measures taken or to be taken

- where available, the conclusions to be drawn from any health surveillance, already undertaken

based on EC Directive 98/24/EC on the protection of the health and safety of workers from the risks related to chemical agents at work 1998

Figure 10.8 Determination and assessment of risk of hazardous chemical reagents

HOW SHOULD HAZARDS BE EVALUATED AND RISKS ASSESSED AND RECORDED?
The Environment, Health and Safety Committee of the Royal Society of Chemistry (UK) have produced a guide entitled 'COSHH in Laboratories'. It was published in 1996, is currently under revision and will subsequently be available on the internet (www.rsc.org). It provides a practical approach which involves hazard evaluation, exposure estimation, risk assessment and control. Guidelines are provided for determining hazard categories as follows; special category (including substances of extreme hazard), high hazard, medium hazard and low hazard. The prime source of information will be the manufacturer's (product)

safety data sheets (MSDS) (see Figure 10.9 continued) and, at St Elsewhere's, all data sheets are filed alphabetically in a central location and are available to all departments. There are now a number of commercial products available on CD ROM that can either replace or supplement such a resource.

Exposure is estimated by using two tables, one for the contribution from inhalation and one the contribution from skin contact. Each table provides a score of 1, 10 or 100 against three factors, (A) the quantity of substance involved, (B) the physical characteristics of the substance and (C) the characteristics of the operation or activity, including the degree of containment provided by the apparatus or equipment used. The scores for each factor are then multiplied together to give a total score for each route of exposure and then total scores used to estimate exposure as low exposure (1, 10 or 100), medium exposure (1,000 or 10,000) or high exposure (100,000 or 1,000,000). An example is given of a task involving the use of 0.5 g of a low volatility liquid in a partially enclosed system which results in a total score of 10 by the inhalation route (low exposure) and 1000 by the dermal route (medium exposure). Use of the tables assumes exposure will be repeated on a daily basis over a prolonged period and an assessor can reduce the exposure assessment if the regular exposure is reduced to say once per week. Finally the general evaluation of risk assessment and control determination can be made in a matrix of hazard against exposure level, to give a risk number. This is on a scale of 1-3 and indicates the conditions under which the work should be undertaken, where 1 = open bench or laboratory, 2 = fume cupboard or other specially vented area and 3 = special facility.

The scheme currently used at St Elsewhere's is demonstrated by the partially completed COSHH assessment form for the assessment of the procedure for the management of a BHM Analyzer [LP-BIO-BHMMan], shown in Figure 10.9. In real life the form is prepared in landscape rather than portrait format.

In addition to the Directive 98/24/EC on the protection of the health and safety of workers from the risks related to chemical agents at work, the IVD Directive (Figure 8.3) requires that devices be manufactured in a manner that 'shall not compromise...the safety and health of users'. The European standard, EN 13641:2002, 'Elimination or reduction of risk of infection related to in vitro diagnostic reagents', provides specific guidance to be followed by the manufacturer. Information provided in the 'hazard and precautions' sections of manufacturer's documentation should be considered as a valuable resource in making risk assessments.

COSHH ASSESSMENT FORM (for use with microorganisms and/or chemicals)

RECORD FILENAME	*MF-GEN-COSHH#LP-BIO-BHMMan*

1 Department	**2 Section**
Biochemistry	*Routine*
3 Assessor name (status or grade)	**4 Status or grade of assessor**
Joanne Jones	*Section supervisor*
5 Date of assessment	**6 Procedure to be assessed**
05/04/02	*Management of BHM Analyzer*

7 Description of procedure

The procedure (together with documentation referenced) details the day to day operation of the BHM Analyzer (for manufacturer's details see equipment database) together with maintenance, servicing and decontamination procedures. It is an open, discrete multichannel analyzer that analyses samples of serum/plasma (from primary blood tubes), CSF and diluted urine for 32 different analytes (see information data sheets for details). COSHH assessment of individual tests is done against laboratory instruction sheets [LI-BIO-BHMGluc] etc.

8 Personnel

It is operated by state registered staff and medical laboratory aides under supervision. All staff wear laboratory coats and gloves.

9. Services and premises (including any miscellaneous potential hazard)

The equipment is free standing with adequate space for its operation. The laboratory has air conditioning. Electrical, water and data services are from the roof space and drainage through a floor grid.

10. Storage of consumable IVDs (including any special precautions)

All consumable IVDs are pre-packaged and stored in a refrigerator at 4°C.

11. Disposal of waste

Clinical waste is disposed of according to Trust procedures and reagent waste through a flushed drainage system.

12 Precautions required (tick appropriate boxes)

Open bench with 'standard precautions'	☐	Gloves (state type)	☐
Safety cabinet Class I	☐	Face/eye protection (state type)	☐
Safety cabinet Class II	☐	Respiratory protection (state type)	☐
Safety cabinet Class III	☐	Stated other protection required:	
Fume cupboard	☐		

based on material provided by the Public Health Laboratory Service (PHLS) UK

Figure 10.9 Partially completed COSHH assessment form

COSHH ASSESSMENT FORM – ASSESSMENT SECTION

PART A: For chemicals in category 'High', 'Medium' or 'Low'

Name of chemical	MSDS YES/NO	Inhalation/ Skin contact	Hazard category			Exposure estimate			Risk No.
			High	Medium	Low	High	Medium	Low	
			☐	☐	☐	☐	☐	☐	
			☐	☐	☐	☐	☐	☐	
			☐	☐	☐	☐	☐	☐	
			☐	☐	☐	☐	☐	☐	

PART B: For microorganisms

Name of organism	ACDP category	Elevation of containment level if appropriate	Reason for elevation

PART C: For extremely toxic substances (e.g. carcinogens, requiring special containment facilities)

Name of agent	Nature of hazard	Personnel using the substance

APPROVAL	NAME	SIGNATURE	DATE
Supervisor			
Safety Officer			
Head of Department			

based on material provided by the Public Health Laboratory Service (PHLS) UK

Figure 10.9 continued, Partially completed COSHH assessment form

For biological agents, the equivalent to the EC directive 98/24/EC for risks related to chemical agents is 90/679/EEC entitled 'Protection of staff from risks related to exposure to biological agents at work'. In Figure 10.9 continued, Part B for Microorganisms, refers to 'ACDP category'. This is the hazard grouping on a scale of 1-4 assigned to particular microorganisms by the Advisory Group on Dangerous Pathogens in the UK. Once the grouping has been determined then the level of containment and safety practice follows.

WHAT TO DO WITH THE INFORMATION FROM THE RISK ASSESSMENT?
In the absence of any specific advice, the view taken at St Elsewhere's is that where the risk assessment requires specific precautions, they shall be detailed in the particular procedure in a panel immediately following the contents page. However, a major emphasis is put on practical training and when a member of staff is introduced to a new procedure the contents of this panel and, if appropriate, the risk assessment record associated with this procedure are discussed. If manufacturer's documentation is to be used then the 'hazards and precautions' sections is discussed. An example of a panel used at St Elsewhere's is shown in Figure 10.10. The issue of how to advise on first aid measures is not entirely resolved and all staff at whatever level are advised to seek advice from a more senior person if in any doubt about the appropriate action to be taken.

HAZARDS and PRECAUTIONS

Substance	Hazards	Precautions/containment regime	First aid code*
Alcian Blue	Blue powder, may cause skin and eye irritation, harmful by inhalation, ingestion, or skin absorption	Avoid contact and inhalation, wear gloves and goggles while preparing stain/open laboratory	A1, B,C,D
Acetic acid (conc)	Colourless liquid, toxic, strongly corrosive, causes serious burns, lachrymator	Wear safety goggles and protective gloves and dispense from stock container/fume cupboard	A1, B,C,D

* **A1** Ingestion, wash mouth thoroughly with water in severe cases obtain medical attention

A2 Ingestion, wash mouth thoroughly with water and give plenty to drink. Seek medical help

B Eye contact, irrigate thoroughly with water for at least ten minutes

C Skin contact, wash off skin thoroughly with water

D Inhalation, remove to fresh air. If severe call a physician

Figure 10.10 Hazards and precautions panel from a laboratory procedure

PRACTICAL APPROACHES TO THE PREPARATION OF EXAMINATION PROCEDURES

There is much advice in the literature on how to prepare examination procedures and for many laboratories it remains a major part of preparing for accreditation. The huge amount of work involved in the in-house preparation of individual procedures led the staff at St Elsewhere's, in common with an increasing number of other laboratories, to re-examine their approach. The re-examination was also driven by the consideration (discussed in Chapter 8), that if an IVD is not used in conformance with the manufacturer's instructions then the liability for malfunction passes from the manufacturer or supplier to the user. This makes it desirable to use manufacturer's information unchanged wherever possible.

In order to determine the best approach it is important to ask the question, 'What is the purpose of the procedure (LP-) and its associated documentation such as working instructions (LI-) and the forms (LF-) used to create records?'. Clearly, the primary purpose is to ensure the proper conduct of the examination or process envisaged and to provide information with which to train and assess the competence of staff. A secondary, but important purpose, is to enable records to be created that allow the reconstruction, as far as is practicable, of any examination or process that has been found to produce nonconformities.

In the author's experience there are some 'general rules' that can be usefully applied (Figure 10.11). These rules apply as much to the preparation of management, clinical and quality procedures as they do to pre-examination, examination and post-examination procedures.

1. Examine the process involved and prepare a flow chart of the practical steps involved.

2. Identify the procedures, instructions and forms currently in use to conduct the process.

3. Determine the **minimum** number of procedures, instructions and forms required to conduct the process.

4. Determine what manufacturer's or other material is available to assist the conduct of the process.

5. If possible create a 'framework' procedure that will allow **maximum** use of manufacturer's or other material and require the **minimum** amount of effort from the laboratory.

6. Trial the documentation **even if it is not perfect** and then review it with all the people who have to use it **as soon as possible.**

Figure 10.11 General rules for the preparation of procedures, instructions and forms

The next section gives different scenarios where these general rules have been tried. The starting point is different for each scenario.

SCENARIO 1
A multichannel analyzer doing assays for three departments

At St Elsewhere's hospital, as a special exercise arising from the 'annual management review', it was decided to to look at a range of quantitative examinations (tests) being done in Biochemistry, Haematology and Microbiology to determine whether some rationalization could take place.

In addition to a wide range of tests being done in Biochemistry on two multichannel instruments, it was established that on three further instruments (two in Biochemistry and one in Microbiology) therapeutic drug assays were being performed and on a sixth instrument in Microbiology, tests related to infectious disease and on a seventh (in Haematology), haematinic assays were being undertaken.

It was decided to replace one of the multichannel instruments in Biochemistry and the remaining six instruments with two BHM Analyzers (BHM = Biochemistry/Haematology and Microbiology). Both were to be situated in the joint Biochemistry/Haematology space and staff from all three departments would use the instruments after appropriate training. All appropriate assays would be done on a 24 hour/7 day per week basis. Biochemistry personnel were asked to devise an approach to documentation.

Following the 'general rules' (Figure 10.11) it was decided that STEP 1 was self explanatory and STEP 2 was not applicable. After consideration of STEPS 3 and 4 it was decided that the manufacturer's Reference Manual met the requirements set out in EN 591:2001 (Figure 8.7) and that the manufacturer's Assay Manual met the requirements set out in EN 375:2001, 'Information supplied by the manufacturer with in vitro diagnostic reagents for professional use' (Figure 10.7) and that together both would fulfil the requirements of ISO 15189:2002 (Figure 10.6).

It was decided that the Reference Manual and the Assay Manual would therefore be registered as controlled documents, [LP-BIO-BHMHnbk] and [LP-BIO-BHMAssy]. Latest versions of manufacturer's calibrator and quality control information sheets (regarded as records) would be dated and kept in a clearly labelled hardback folder. All other records are kept in electronic format on the BHM analyzers and appropriate backup procedures for these records instigated.

As STEP 5, it was decided that a framework procedure, [LP-BIO-BHMMan] would be written to provide reference to appropriate sections of the manufacturer's manuals. A diagram was created to represent these decisions (Figure 10.12). The procedure is a controlled document with the same header material that is used throughout the laboratory (see Figure 4.2 for an example).

The *Contents* are preceded by *Hazards and precautions* information, *0 Introduction*, *1 Pre-examination* process with reference to the Users Handbook, [PD-GEN-UserHbk], *2 Examination process* with reference to two in-house instruction sheets for starting up and shutting down the analyzer to standby [LI-BIO-BHMStrt] and [LI-BIO-BHMStby]. These are controlled documents and displayed by the analyzer for day to day use. Reference is also made to the quality procedure for external quality assessment [QP-BIO-EQA] and finally, section *3 Post-examination process* providing in-house information on reference values, authorization and reporting [LP-BIO-Report].

STEP 6 will be undertaken after three months and subsequently the documentation will be reviewed on an annual basis in compliance with document control procedures (Chapter 5).

SCENARIO 2
The production of a routine Haematoxylin and Eosin (H and E) stained section.

At St Elsewhere's hospital, the Histopathology Department decided to review its rather ad hoc documentation for the production of an H and E stained section. The publication of professional guidelines proposing that the cut-up of some specimens could be undertaken by trained technologists rather than specialist pathologists required a clarification of responsibilities and the establishment of a 'triage' system. Finally, agreement was being sought between the four Histopathologists on reporting procedures and minimum data sets for reporting.

A working party was established with membership from pathologists and technologists and it was agreed to ask the quality manager to undertake STEP 1 and produce a process diagram of the practical steps involved and relate them to the appropriate clauses of the 'Ideal Standard'. After much discussion the diagram shown in Figure 10.13 was agreed.

Management of the BHM Analyzers [LP-BIO-BHMMan]

Hazards and precautions
Contents
0 Introduction
  0.1 Purpose and scope
  0.2 Responsibility
  0.3 References
  0.4 Definitions
  0.5 Documentation

1 Pre-examination process   [PD-GEN-UserHbk]
  1.1 Patient preparation
  1.2 Primary blood samples
  1.3 Urine samples
  1.4 Cerebral spinal fluid

2 Examination process
  2.1 System principles*
  2.2 System overview*
  2.3 User interface facility*
  2.4 Operating the system*
    2.4.1 Start up from standby* [LI-BIO-BHMStrt]
    2.4.3 Shutdown to standby* [LI-BIO-BHMStby]
  2.5 Calibration*
  2.6 Internal quality control*
  2.7 External quality assessment [QP-BIO-EQA]
  2.8 Methodology**
    2.8.1 Biochemistry examinations**
    2.8.2 Haematology examinations**
    2.8.3 Microbiology examinations**
  2.9 Maintenance*
  2.10 System troubleshooting*
  2.11 Assay troubleshooting*
  2.12 Setup*
  2.13 Validation of results

3 Post-examination process
  3.1 Reference values [PD-GEN-UserHbk]
  3.2 Authorization of reports [LP-BIO-Report]
  3.3 Reporting and interpretative comments

*Manufacturer's Reference Manual (Handbook)
[LP-BIO-BHMHnbk]

File labelled **Manufacturer's calibrator information sheets**
(current versions)

File labelled **Manufacturer's quality control information sheets**
(current versions)

**Manufacturer's Assay Manual
[LP-BIO-BHMHnbk]

Electronic records held on the analyzer

- Patients results, run numbers and dates
- Internal quality control and calibration
  results, change of batch data and dates
- Reagent change of batch data and dates
- External quality assessment programme
  results and dates

Figure 10.12 SCENARIO 1 – Documentation for the BHM Analyzer

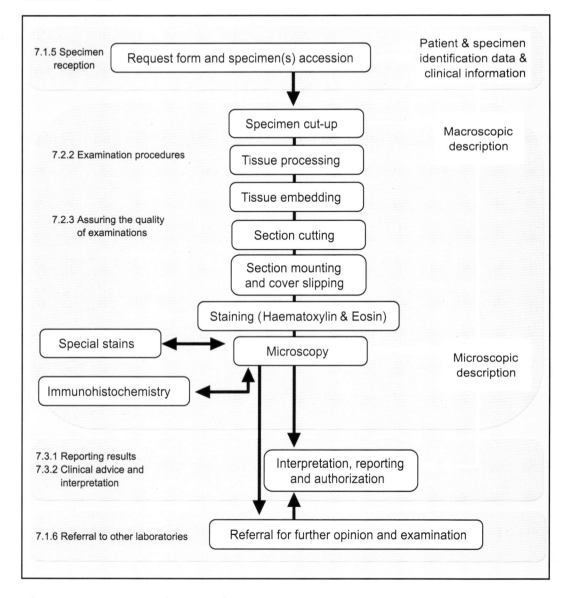

Figure 10.13 Process diagram for a routine H and E stained section

In STEPS 2 and 3, the working party collected together all the existing documentation and determined that only three procedures were required; a framework procedure for production of routine H and E stained sections [LP-HIS-RoutH&E], a separate procedure for immunohistochemistry [LP-HIS-ImmHist] and the quality procedure for participation in external quality assessment schemes [QP-

HIS-EQA] that was already in existence. It was decided to create 'protocols for cut-up' [LI-HIS-CutupXY], 'laboratory instructions for special stains' [LI-HIS-StainXY]and 'protocols for reporting' [LI-HIS-ReptXY] and register them all as laboratory instructions in Q-pulse (LI-HIS-) and keep them in labelled hard-backed files for easy day to day access.

STEP 4 involved examining the available manufacturer's instructions for the equipment for tissue processing and embedding, section cutting and mounting and microscopy and register them as laboratory procedures [LP-HIS-]. Finally, it was agreed to keep in a labelled file, manufacturer's reagent information fact sheets for all the stains in use. STEP 5 involved writing the framework procedure and creating the diagram shown in Figure 10.14 to represent all these decisions. The process diagram (Figure 10.13) and this diagram are used within the frame-work procedure on the basis that 'two diagrams are worth two thousand words'. STEP 6 will involve an initial review at six months and from then on annually in compliance with document control procedures (Chapter 5). The documents used to review procedures for cut-up and reporting, published by the CAP, RCPath UK and NPAAC are cited in Appendix 2 Further reading.

The European standard, EN 12376:1999, 'In vitro diagnostic medical devices – Information provided by the manufacturer with in vitro diagnostic reagents for staining in biology' specifies 'requirements for the information supplied by the manufacturer'. It applies to producers, suppliers and vendors of dyes, stains, chromogenic and other reagents used for staining in biology. It is seen as addi-tional to, and not replacing, information given in EN 375:2001 (Figure 10.7). Annex A, gives examples of the way in which information might be provided by the manufacturer, and includes the Methyl green – Pyronin Y stain, the Feulgen-Schiff reaction, immunohistochemical demonstration of oestrogen recepters and flow cytometric demonstration of T-cells. The standard has application to other disciplines of pathology e.g. stains used for visualization of proteins in elec-trophoresis etc.

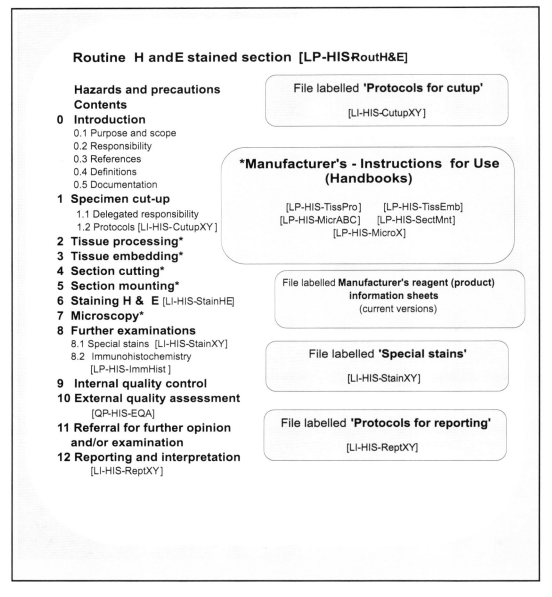

Routine H andE stained section [LP-HISRoutH&E]

Hazards and precautions
Contents
0 Introduction
 0.1 Purpose and scope
 0.2 Responsibility
 0.3 References
 0.4 Definitions
 0.5 Documentation
1 Specimen cut-up
 1.1 Delegated responsibility
 1.2 Protocols [LI-HIS-CutupXY]
2 Tissue processing*
3 Tissue embedding*
4 Section cutting*
5 Section mounting*
6 Staining H & E [LI-HIS-StainHE]
7 Microscopy*
8 Further examinations
 8.1 Special stains [LI-HIS-StainXY]
 8.2 Immunohistochemistry
  [LP-HIS-ImmHist]
9 Internal quality control
10 External quality assessment
 [QP-HIS-EQA]
11 Referral for further opinion
 and/or examination
12 Reporting and interpretation
 [LI-HIS-ReptXY]

File labelled **'Protocols for cutup'**

[LI-HIS-CutupXY]

***Manufacturer's - Instructions for Use**
(Handbooks)

[LP-HIS-TissPro]   [LP-HIS-TissEmb]
[LP-HIS-MicrABC]   [LP-HIS-SectMnt]
[LP-HIS-MicroX]

File labelled **Manufacturer's reagent (product)**
information sheets
(current versions)

File labelled **'Special stains'**

[LI-HIS-StainXY]

File labelled **'Protocols for reporting'**

[LI-HIS-ReptXY]

Figure 10.14 SCENARIO 2 – Documentation for a routine H & E stained section

The headings used in Annex A in relation to the Feulgen-Schiff reaction are shown in Figure 10.15. When the quality of the information provided by the manufacturer meets the standard in this example it could be used to replace or create the laboratory instructions for special stains [LI-HIS-SpStXYZ] (see Figure 10.14).

Feulgen-Schiff reaction

Pararosaniline dye	**Intended use of the Feulgen-Schiff reaction**
Product name	Type(s) of material
Cautionary statement	Handling and treatment before staining
Composition	Details of the procedure used by the manufacturer to test the reactivity of the chromogenic reagent
Wavelength of maximum absorption of dye solution	*Pararosaniline-Schiff reagent*
Thin layer chromatography	*Rinsing solution*
Handling and storage	*Staining procedure*
	Results expected with the recommended type(s) of material

based on Annex A (informative) EN 12376:1999 In vitro diagnostic medical devices - Information supplied by the manufacturer with the in vitro diagnostic reagents for staining in biology

---

Figure 10.15 Headings for the Feulgen-Schiff reaction

SCENARIO 3
Routine investigation of urine samples in Microbiology

At St Elsewhere's Hospital, due to retirements, two new Microbiologists have been appointed who, unlike the previous incumbents, came from the Public Health Laboratory Service (currently the PHLS but from April 2003 to be known as the Health Protection Agency). In their previous employments they were used to the Standard Operating Procedures (SOPs) produced by the PHLS. A further stimulus to a re-evaluation of documentation was that the neighbouring hospitals, with which St Elsewhere's are to co-operate in the near future, were already investigating the use of PHLS SOPs.

In STEPS 1-3, a joint working party with membership from all three hospitals was established. After the first meeting it was decided, a) to ask the Chief Technologists and the Quality Manager from St Elsewhere's (the only Quality Manager currently in post) to undertake a survey of all documentation currently in place for all examinations in relation to the SOPs produced by the PHLS and b) for the working group to examine the PHLS SOP for 'Investigation of Urine' (PHLS B.SOP.41) to see whether it met current requirements and to determine the steps needed to bring such documentation into practical use and into the document control system.

It was quickly decided that PHLS B.SOP.41 was very comprehensive, but that unlike some SOPs from the PHLS, it did not have a section on quality assurance (internal quality control and external quality assessment), or much information on the limitations of the method. Participation in external quality assessment schemes was already covered in [QP-MIC-EQA]. Correspondence with the PHLS revealed that a programme of continuing revision was in place and that the website invites registration for this update service.

It was agreed that in general, PHLS SOPs should be used subject to the actions shown in Figure 10.16 being implemented. This sequence of action could equally be applied to material from any outside source.

---

1. The procedure (in this case PHLS B.SOP.41) should be examined in detail to see whether it fits current practice in the laboratory.

2. Any modifications required to the procedure to fit current practice should be made and a brief record made of these changes in a new section, **7 Changes for local practice.**

3. The procedure should then be reformatted by removing the PHLS footer information and adding the St Elsewhere's header (see Chapter 5), changing the title page and removing the amendment procedure page.

4. The procedure should then be registered as a draft document [LP-MI-BSOP41], to retain its relationship with PHLS B.SOP.41 and be subject to document control procedures (see Figure 5.8).

5. When a revised PHLS B.SOP.41 is published, it would be examined as in step 1 (above) and a decision made as to whether to proceed with steps 2-4, or retain the original procedure.

Figure 10.16 Action to be taken to adopt procedures/documents from an outside source

New sections, 4.0a Internal quality control, and 4.0b External quality assessment, were added, the numbering chosen to avoid disturbing the sequencing of numbering in order to save unnecessary work. The section on internal quality control will be guided by information in European Standard EN 12322:1999, 'In vitro diagnostic medical devices – Culture media for microbiology – Performance criteria for culture media'. The scope of the standard states that 'it specifies requirements for the performance of culture media' and is applicable to: a) commercial organizations distributing media to microbiological laboratories in ready to use form, as dehydrated media or as semi-finished media, b) non-commercial organizations that distribute media to satellite locations and c) laboratories that prepare culture media for their own use. The section on external quality assessment will provide details of membership of EQA schemes and refer to the procedure for participation in external quality assessment [QP-MIC-EQA].

In pursuit of STEP 4 scrutiny of manufacturer's information (see Figure 8.7) revealed that the manufacturer's handbooks/instructions for use, on incubators and microscopes used in urine investigation should be registered in the document control system. All incubators, refrigerators etc used throughout pathology are subject to a procedure for temperature monitoring [LP-GEN-ManTemp] and appropriate reference is made in the procedure to the forms upon which records of monitoring etc. should be kept. STEP 5 illustrates the approach taken (Figure 10.17). STEP 6 will involve an initial review at six months and from then on, annually in compliance with document control procedures (Chapter 5).

ASSURING THE QUALITY OF EXAMINATIONS
'Ideal Standard' clause 7.2.3 Ensuring the quality of examinations

INTRODUCTION
Inspection of Figure 10.1 will show that clause 7.2.3 of the 'Ideal Standard' is entitled 'Assuring the quality of examinations', in order to correspond to the clauses of ISO 15189:2002 and ISO 17025:1999 that begin *'Assuring the quality...'*. However, there is an important distinction to be drawn between those activities which *ensure* on a day to day basis the quality of examinations and those which contribute to the broader concept of *assuring* the quality of examinations.

A number of activities play a major part, on a 'day to day' basis, in ensuring the quality of an examination (a measurement or observation). These include calibration (where applicable), and having proper control of reagents. Changes in calibration data can sound alarm bells, but it is significant deviations in the results from internal quality control material, acting as surrogates for patient samples, that prevent the wrong result from being authorized and reported.

Investigation of Urine [LP- MIC-BSOP41] based on PHLS B.SOP.41

Amendment procedure   (page to be removed)

Introduction

    Clinical manifestations of UTI

    Incidence of UTI

    Organisms

    Specimen collection

    Diagnosis of UTI

    Significant Bacteriuria

    Additional non-culture screening methods for UTI

    Other urine investigations

> **Manufacturer's - Instructions for Use (Handbooks)**
> Incubators, refrigerators, microscopes etc

1.0 Safety consideration

    1.1 Specimen collection

    1.2 Specimen transport and storage

    1.3 Specimen processing

> File labelled **Manufacturer's reagent (product) information sheets**
> (current versions)

2.0 Specimen collection

    2.1 Optimal time of specimen collection

    2.2 Correct specimen type and methods of collection

    2.3 Adequate quantity and appropriate number of specimens

3.0 Specimen transport and storage

    3.1 Time between specimen collection and processing

    3.2 Special considerations to minimise deterioration

4.0 Specimen processing

    4.1 Test selection

    4.2 Appearance

    4.3 Microscopy or alternative screening method

    4.4 Culture and investigation

    4.5 Identification

    4.6 Susceptibility testing

    4.0a Internal quality control

    4.0b External quality assessment [QP-MIC-EQA]

5.0 Reporting procedure

    5.1 Microscopy or alternative screening procedure

    5.2 Susceptibility testing

6.0 Reporting to the CDSC and CSCDC

References

7.0 Changes for local practice

Figure 10.17 SCENARIO 3 – Documentation for a routine urine investigation

Major contributions to assuring the quality of an examination would include evidence of appropriate training of staff (Chapter 6), the selection and validation of equipment (Chapter 8), and participation in external quality assessment schemes and the internal audit of examination processes (Chapter 11). The first two activities can be regarded as making a prospective contribution, and the latter two a retrospective contribution to assuring the quality of an examination. No amount of participation in external quality assessment schemes will stop an erroneous result being reported on the day, but good internal quality control procedures will minimise that risk. Ensuring a correct report as distinct from ensuring a correct result (technical validation) was dealt with under post-examination processes in Chapter 9.

In ISO 17025:1999 (because of the nature of the standard), and in ISO 15189:2002 (in part), the major emphasis is on examinations involving measurement. Emphasis is on use of internal quality control materials and controlling changes in reagents and calibrators that contribute to uncertainty, and on participation in external quality assessment schemes or alternatives.

UNCERTAINTY
In order to ensure the quality of examination procedures it is important to be able to identify and delineate the uncertainties associated with the procedures. Being uncertain about something is defined in common English usage as 'not to be accurately known or predicted' and uncertainty is 'the state of being uncertain'. To be able to understand the causes of uncertainty and to seek to minimise them is the key to to ensuring the quality of examinations. In the ISO publication, 'Guide to the expression of uncertainty in measurement' a distinction is drawn between the general concept of uncertainty (in this case applied to measurements) and uncertainty defined as a 'parameter associated with the result of a measurement, that characterises the dispersion of the values that could be reasonably be attributed to the measurand' (the quantity being measured e.g. amount of a substance or a concentration).

This emphasis is unhelpful to a consideration of examinations that are based on observations, where uncertainty, although not readily definable in terms of dispersion of values, is present and can be minimised by appropriate measures. Interestingly, ISO 15189:2002 focuses on 'uncertainty of results' rather than uncertainty of measurement and details potential contributions to uncertainty, such as sample preparation, sample portion selection, calibrators, reference materials, equipment used, environmental conditions and the influence of changing operators. Many of the factors can be identified as affecting examinations based on observation as well as measurement. At St Elsewhere's, arising from an interdisciplinary working party, a programme of courses has been established to train staff in the identification of all potential contributions to uncertainty, or put another way, sources of nonconformity, in pre-examination, examination and post-examination processes, and to suggest preventative action. It follows the style of the two hour programme for 'Good Housekeeping' audit discussed in Chapter 7, participation is multidisciplinary and uses a form similar to that shown in Figure 7.22.

INTERNAL QUALITY CONTROL

A major part of any examination procedure is the performance of quality control procedures. The term 'quality control' has been misused consistently in the literature over a long period of time, and it is, therefore, important to define the difference between (internal) quality control activities and (external) quality assessment. The latter term is often referred to as external quality control, which it is not, as it does not control the production of examination results on a day to day basis. Figure 10.18 gives a useful definition of quality control which indicates its role and limitations.

(Internal) quality control.....

...is the set of procedures undertaken by the staff of a laboratory for continuously assessing laboratory work and the emergent results, in order to decide whether they are reliable enough to be released (either in support of clinical decision making or for epidemiological or research purposes). Thus quality control procedures have an immediate effect on the laboratory's activities and should actually control, as opposed to merely examining, the laboratory's output.

WHO External Assessment of Health Laboratories (1981)

Figure 10.18   Definition of internal quality control

USE OF QUALITY CONTROL MATERIAL

The use of quality control materials, to monitor the performance of a TSH assay, or to ensure that an agar plate will allow the growth of an organism, are at the core of ensuring the quality of examinations on a day to day basis. The issues for accreditation are three-fold.

Firstly, that the material used is appropriate to the examination being controlled and to the purpose of that examination. For example, that control materials for a TSH assay, have a compatible matrix and analyte concentrations that simulate clinically important levels, and preferably that the source of the material is independent of the manufacturer of the IVD being used in the examination process. Secondly, that criteria are established that allow the detection of aberrant results in a manner that maintains the examination procedure within its required performance characteristics and thirdly, that there is documentary evidence of the results and of any action taken as a result of aberrant results.

CHANGE CONTROL

The concept of 'change control' was first discussed in Chapter 8 in the context of computer systems. In that situation, the aim is to ensure that should any malfunctions appear in the system it is possible to associate them with particular changes in hardware and/or software. The inverse is a fundamental concept in experimental science, that in order to detect significant change in an experimental system, only one variable, for example the temperature, should be changed at a time. In examination procedures, it is the quality control material that is the constant, the indicator of unwanted change or aberrant functioning. Change control in this situation should then follow certain principles, a) that no changes in calibration or reagents should be made at the same time as a change in quality control material, b) there should be an overlap in changes of quality control material and c) ideally only one variable in the examination procedure should be changed at a time, for example, either a set of calibrators or a reagent, but not both at the same time. These changes must be documented either in a manual system or in the 'on board' systems available on many modern analyzers. This documentation is closely related to stock control practices discussed in Chapter 8.

POINT-OF-CARE TESTING

Near patient or point-of-care testing (POCT) has been documented at least since Thomas Willis (1621-1675) wrote of tasting urine to test for glycosuria. Developments in technology, particularly of the so-called dry chemistry over the past fifteen years, have created many opportunities for pathology tests to be performed outside the conventional laboratory. Within a hospital the situations range from urine stick tests in a side room of a ward or blood glucose and glycated haemoglobin measurements in a Diabetic Clinic, to Intensive Care Units with blood gas and electrolyte analysers. In many countries, primary care physicians (general practitioners) will perform an increasing range of POCT examinations.

Leaving aside issues of cost effectiveness and efficacy, the College of American Pathologists left no doubt as to their position on the introduction of POCT, '…quality of patient care is the highest priority. Alternative site testing must not introduce or augment clinically significant errors in the testing process…

Alternative site testing requires adherence to the standards of good laboratory practice, including quality control, quality assurance, proficiency testing and recording of results in the patient's medical record'. It is clear from this statement that point-of-care testing must not be regarded as a special case exempt from standards of practice associated with an accredited laboratory.

For those seeking practical advice the literature on POCT testing is now extensive and a number of key references are cited in Appendix 2 Further reading. Pre-eminent among them is the publication from the American Association of Clinical Chemistry (AACC) on Point-of-Care Testing. This brings together in one place, the analytical principles of POCT, the management issues and case studies of actual or potential applications. Of particular importance to accreditation is the treatment given to management issues such as procurement of equipment, training and certification of staff, supervision of testing, quality control and quality assurance, laboratory management and the economics of POCT.

To assist those preparing a procedure for the management of POCT, the contents of the procedure written by the Joint Working Party on POCT at St Elsewhere's Hospital is shown in Figure 10.19.

---

0 INTRODUCTION
  0.1 Purpose and scope
  0.2 Responsibilities
  0.3 References
  0.4 Definitions
  0.5 Documentation

1 ORGANIZATION AND MANAGEMENT
  1.1 Working Group on POCT
  1.2 Membership
  1.3 Agendas and minutes
  1.4 Frequency of meetings

2 IN VITRO DIAGNOSTIC DEVICES
  2.1 IVD inventory
  2.2 IVD maintenance
  2.3 Stock control and issue of IVDs

3 HAZARDS AND PRECAUTIONS

4 TRAINING AND CERTIFICATION
  4.1 Trainers
  4.2 Training courses
  4.3 Register of certified users

5 DOCUMENTATION
  5.1 Procedures, working instructions and forms
  5.2 Manufacturer's information
  5.3 Patient's records
  5.4 Quality records

6 ASSURING THE QUALITY OF POCT
  6.1 Internal quality control
  6.2 External quality assessment
  6.3 Internal quality audit

7 INTERPRETATION AND COMMUNICATION OF RESULTS

Figure 10.19 Procedure for the management of POCT [LP-GEN-POCT]

Chapter 11

Evaluation and continual improvement

INTRODUCTION

'Ideal Standard' clause 8 Evaluation and continual improvement

The title of this chapter has been chosen to try to convey the idea that any laboratory should be constantly evaluating its activities and seeking to continually maintain and improve quality. The title of the equivalent clause in ISO 9001:2000, clause 8 *'Measurement, analysis and improvement'*, is confusing to laboratory personnel, who more readily associate 'measurement and analysis' with examination procedures than with the quality process. The relationship between the clauses of the 'Ideal Standard' and the ISO 9001:2000, ISO 17025:1999 and ISO 15189:2002 are shown in Appendix 1. An important source of information for this chapter is ISO 9004:2000 'QMS – Guidelines for performance improvements'. Its scope makes it clear that 'it provides guidelines beyond the requirements given in ISO 9001:2000 in order to consider both the effectiveness and efficiency of a QMS and consequently the potential for improvement of the performance of an organization'. This standard together with ISO 9000:2000, ISO 9001:2000 (see Figure 2.9) ISO 17025:1999 and ISO 15189:2002 should be on the desk of every quality manager working in a medical laboratory.

Evaluation and continual improvement could be regarded as synonymous with quality assurance, but it seems increasingly uncertain what is meant by the term 'quality assurance'. The difficulty seems to arise from the meanings of the words 'assure' and 'ensure'. To try to ensure the quality of something is 'to make sure or certain' of its quality, whereas to assure 'to give confidence to oneself or others' seems a relatively impotent activity if you view it from the point of view of the user clinician.

Donabedian (see Appendix 2, Further reading), defined 'quality assurance' in relation to healthcare as 'the managed process whereby the comparison of care against predetermined standards is guaranteed to lead to action to implement changes, and ensuring that these have produced the desired improvement'. That in itself seems a useful and acceptable definition, but Donabedian himself did not particularly like the term quality assurance, regarding it as 'too optimistic a term' and spoke more about evaluation and assessment in his seminal works on quality in healthcare. Figure 11.1 illustrates the inter-connectivity of the different aspects of evaluation and quality improvement as detailed in Clause 8 of the 'Ideal Standard'.

The LABORATORY (the Organization)...

...seeks to constantly evaluate all aspects of performance by establishing procedures...

8.1 General

8.2 Internal Audit

... that use...

...to make an...

8.2.1 Assessment of user satisfaction and complaints

...and...

8.2.2 Internal audit of the quality management system

...and...

8.2.3 Internal audit of examination processes

...together with the results of...

8.3 External audit

...from...

8.3.1 External quality assessment programmes

...and...

8.3.2 External reviews

...and the investigation of...

8.4 Nonconforming examinations

...to contribute to....

8.5 Improvement

...and creates a culture of ...

8.5.1 Continual improvement

...that provides for...

8.5.2 Corrective action

...and...

8.5.3 Preventive action

Figure 11.1 Clause 8 of the 'Ideal Standard' – Evaluation and quality improvement

The opening sections of this chapter deal with the role of internal audit and external assessments in detecting nonconformity in the QMS and in examination procedures themselves. The role of continual improvement is dealt with in relation to a concept of circles of continual improvement and to the central role of management review.

GENERAL
'Ideal Standard' clause 8.1 General

The overall aim of evaluation and quality improvement in a medical laboratory is to continue to meet the needs and requirements of users. A translation of ISO 9001:2000, clause 8.1 *'General'* for the laboratory requires that, it plans and implements activity that enables it to demonstrate the conformity of the results of examination procedures, the proper functioning of the QMS and provides evidence of continual improvement.

DEFINITIONS
In this book the author has tried to avoid the use of unfamiliar terms, but in the area of evaluation and improvement certain terms improve communication and these are given in Figure 11.2.

---

audit
systematic, independent and documented process for obtaining audit evidence and evaluating it objectively to determine the extent to which audit criteria are fulfilled

nonconformity
non-fulfillment of a requirement

corrective action
action taken to eliminate the cause of a detected nonconformity or other undesirable situation

preventive action
action taken to eliminate the cause of a potential nonconformity or other undesirable potential situation

continual improvement
re-occuring activity to increase the ability to fulfil requirements

ISO 9000:2000 Quality management systems – Fundamentals and vocabulary

---

Figure 11.2 Definitions in relation to evaluation and quality improvement

A *nonconformity* can arise in two distinct ways. Firstly, from an (reactive) *audit* resulting from a problem in the conduct of a process, leading to the need for *corrective* and/or *preventive action* and thus contributing to the maintenance of quality or to *continual improvement*. Or secondly, a proactive *audit* produces a *nonconformity* that again requires *corrective* and/or *preventive action*, thus contributing to the maintenance of quality or to *continual improvement*.

An example of the first situation, occurred in St Elsewhere's Biochemistry department. An inspection of the first results from a new batch of quality control material being introduced on the BHM analyzer (change control) showed that results at all three levels for each analyte were approximately 20% lower than expected *(a nonconformity)*. Investigation *(an audit)*, revealed that although the freeze dried material had been reconstituted with 5 ml of reconstituting fluid as per the documented procedure, the manufacturer had changed the reconstitution volume from 5 ml to 4 ml without sending out a notice to this effect. All vials wrongly reconstituted were immediately removed *(corrective action)*. Following this incident all personnel involved had the matter drawn to their attention and the procedure was altered and an adverse incident report dispatched to the Medical Devices Agency UK, with a copy to the manufacturer *(preventive action)*. These actions contribute to ensuring the quality of examinations, *(continual improvement)*. An example of a proactive audit would be a 'good housekeeping audit' and such audits are at the core of maintaining a programme of continual improvement.

TYPES OF AUDIT
The ISO definition of audit is shown in Figure 11.2. Three different types of audit can usefully be distinguished. The first, is an *internal audit* conducted by the laboratory itself (or occasionally on behalf of a laboratory by an outside auditor) on some aspect of laboratory activity such as the accuracy of transcription of data from a request form into the LIS, or whether all members of staff have up to date job descriptions. The second, is *external audit* (sometimes termed assessments) conducted by some person or bodies interested in the organization such as a purchasing authority or by external independent organizations such CPA(UK)Ltd or a regulatory authority. A third type of audit, not shown in orthodox classifications, is *co-operative audit* conducted between the laboratory and another party for mutual benefit. Examples of co-operative audit are clinical audit or customer satisfaction surveys and bench marking activities. Schemes for external quality assessment that are run on a primarily educational basis can in some senses be regarded as cooperative audit, but in this text they are discussed under external audit. Audits as we have seen earlier provide an important mechanism for the detection and investigation of nonconformity. Later in the chapter methods of audit are discussed.

MANAGEMENT OF EVALUATION AND CONTINUAL IMPROVEMENT

At St Elsewhere's the management of evaluation and continual improvement activity is the prime remit of the Quality Manager (see Figure 4.8) and he works with the Quality and Accreditation (Q&A) Committee in Pathology and reports directly to the Director of Pathology (see Figure 4.16). All groups, medical, scientific, technical, administrative and service staff are represented on the Q&A committee. In each department there is a quality group that reports to the Q&A committee These groups set departmental standards, review results from external quality assessment schemes, co-ordinate and supervise day to day quality control activities, and undertake clinical audit. As with the organization and management of computing, it is important that each discipline has a quality co-ordinator who liaises closely with the quality manager.

Evaluation and continual improvement activity makes a major input into the annual management review and the Quality Manager's role in that activity is discussed later in the chapter. The content of the procedure for the management of evaluation and continual improvement [QP-GEN-Eval&CI] is shown in Figure 11.3. Audit and nonconformities (called nonconformance in Q-Pulse) are managed through the Gael Quality product, Q-Pulse. The Q-Pulse manual is registered in the document control system (Figure 5.13). Its use and reference to it means that [QP-GEN-Eval&CI] is only 8 pages in length and serves as a framework procedure.

INTERNAL AUDIT

'Ideal Standard' clause 8.2 Internal audit

In January 1996, the European Co-operation for Accreditation (EA) published a valuable document EA-4/04 'Internal Audits and Management Review for laboratories' (original code EAL-G3). Its intention is to provide assistance to laboratories seeking to perform internal audits and use them as input to management reviews. Although the references throughout the guide are to EN 45001 and ISO Guide 25 (now replaced by ISO 17025:1999) and although it was formally withdrawn in October 2001, its content is still very valuable (see Figure 11.4).

Procedure for the management of evaluation and continual improvement [QP-GEN-Eval&CI]

0 Introduction
1 Quality and accreditation committee
    1.1 Chairperson, deputy chairperson and secretary
    1.2 Membership and co-option
    1.3 Responsibilities of members
    1.4 Quality manager
2 Departmental quality groups
3 Frequency, agenda and minutes of meetings*
4 Communications*
5 Internal audit*
    5.1 User satisfaction and complaints*
        (including clinical audit [QP-GEN-ClinAud]
    5.2 Staff suggestions*
    5.3 Quality management system*
    5.4 Examination processes*
    5.5 Self assessment*
6 External audit*
    6.1 External quality assessment schemes [QP-XXX-EQA]
    6.2 External assessments*
7 Nonconforming examinations*
8 Quality improvement*
    8.1 Continual improvement
    8.2 Registrationof nonconformity*
    8.3 Corrective action*
    8.4 Preventative action*

***Q-Pulse Version 4 Users Manual**

[MP-GEN-QPULSE4]

Q-Pulse files

Keep audit schedules and checklists and records of audit reports and nonconformities

Track progress on nonconformities and record corrective and preventative action

Figure 11.3 Contents of the procedure for the management of evaluation and continual improvement [QP-GEN-Eval&CI]

METHODS OF AUDIT

Two methods of internal audit, horizontal and vertical are defined in EA-4/04 and at St Elsewhere's, two further methods are used, witness audit and self assessment. Figure 11.5 shows the relationship between horizontal, vertical and witness audits in relation to the individual elements of a process. It shows a linear process with four separate elements (A-D) with inputs and outputs. This could represent two scenarios, the first, in relation to the conduct of examinations. The separate elements might be pre-examination (A and B), examination (C) and post-examination (D). A second scenario, might represent the preparation (A), authorization (B), issue and distribution (C) and review (D) elements of a document preparation and control process (Figure 5.8).

1	Introduction	8	Organization of management reviews
2	Terminology		
		9	Objectives of management reviews
3	Objectives of internal audits		
		10	Planning and implementation of management reviews
4	Organization of internal audits		
5	Planning of internal audits	11	Records of management reviews
6	Implementation of internal audits	12	References
7	Documentation of internal audits		

Figure 11.4 Content of EA-4/04, 'Internal audits and management review for laboratories'

In the first scenario, a vertical audit would involve selecting a single request form and its associated sample *(the input)* and following through every element of the process (A-D) until the report is produced *(the output)*. A horizontal audit would select one element of the process (D), for example the report, and examine a number of reports to see for example, whether appropriate interpretative comments and/or followup of abnormal results had been provided. A witness audit of the examination element (C) would observe a person or group of people carrying out the particular task, firstly to ensure that what is being done reflects what is described in the procedure and secondly, that the person(s) carrying out the examination has a good understanding of all aspects of the procedure.

In the second scenario a vertical audit would involve selecting a particular document to check that all elements (A-D) in its preparation and control had been completed according to the procedure [MP-GEN-DocCtrl] (Figure 5.7). A horizontal audit of the review element might check to see that all management forms had been reviewed within the preset interval for review. A witness audit, such as observing the proper use of a document control package (e.g. Q-pulse) would be possible in the second scenario, but is more commonly used in pre-examination and examination processes.

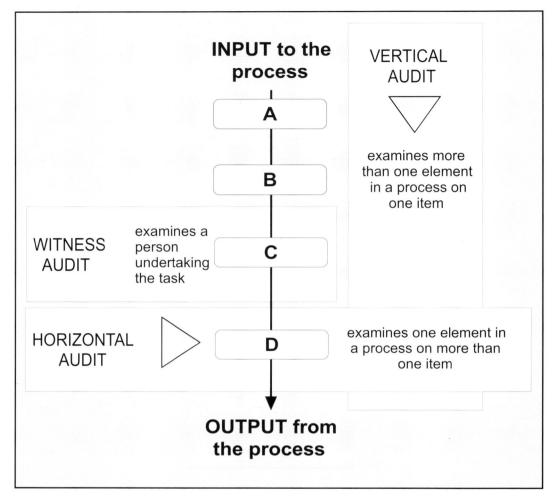

Figure 11.5 Methods of audit

ISO 9004:2000 describes self assessment as 'a careful evaluation, usually performed by the organization's own management, that results in an opinion or judgement of the effectiveness and efficiency of an organization and the maturity of the quality management system'. Although categorised in this text as an approach to audit it is broader in concept, depending more on opinion or judgement than upon predetermined audit criteria, it seeks for example, to form a view on such questions as 'How does laboratory management demonstrate its leadership, commitment and involvement?', 'How does the organization ensure that statutory and regulatory requirements have been considered?'. Annex A of ISO 9004:2000 provides valuable guidelines for self assessment and includes a list of 27 questions which relate to the requirements for all aspects of a QMS set out in

ISO 9001:2000. An example of self assessment is the contribution it can make in preparation for an annual joint review (Figure 6.12). In a sense 'staff suggestions', discussed later in the chapter can also be a form of self assesssment.

AUDIT PROCEDURE

The problem of conducting audits without a computer package is not insurmountable, but the adequate tracking of nonconformities and the corrective or preventive action consequent upon their discovery is not easy.

AUDIT SCHEDULE FORM

RECORD FILENAME		QF-GEN-AudSch#H&S2002

1 Type of audit calender	2 Date of preparation	3 Year
Health and safety	03 September 2001	2002

Audit topic	Jan	Feb	Mar	Apr	Jun	Jul	Aug	Sep	Oct	Nov	Dec
Good housekeeping	AUDIT 03/01/02 J Q NC	CHECK 03/02/02 J Q				AUDIT					
Waste disposal		AUDIT 10/02/02 J Q NC	CHECK				AUDIT				
Protective clothing			AUDIT 03/03/02 J Q					AUDIT			

Progress in the audit calender is recorded as below

Indicates the month of the audit	AUDIT	Indicates the need for check audit	CHECK
Indicates the date completed and by whom (NC indicates nonconformities recorded)	AUDIT 03/03/02 J Q NC	Indicates the date the check audit was completed and nonconformities discharged	CHECK 03/03/02 J Q

Figure 11.6 An audit schedule

The procedure contents shown in Figure 11.4 indicate the steps in a successful audit programme; planning (scheduling audits), implementation (deciding what should be audited and conducting the audit), and documentation (recording the findings and in particular the items that give rise to nonconformities).

Until recently at St Elsewhere's audits were conducted using an entirely paper based system and examples of the forms used will illustrate the process (Figures 11.9, 11.11 and 11.12). Audits were scheduled using the form shown in Figure 11.6. This audit calender, plan or schedule can be created in a spreadsheet or as a table in a word processing package.

1.0 Creating an audit schedule

    1.1 Choose the type of audit calender (i.e. Internal audit, Health and safety or create title

    1.2 What would you like to audit?
- by area of the standard
- by department
- by supplier
- by documentation

    1.3 Select the audit title
- 'Ideal Standard' Clause 6.5 Management of data and information systems
- Haematology
- named supplier/manufacturer
- all [MP-GEN-] procedures

    1.4 Schedule the date(s) of the audit

    1.5 Select the auditor, auditee and department

2.0 Preparing for an audit (this function notifies staff of an impending audit)

3.0 Preparing an audit checklist

    3.1 Create a master list of audit questions

    3.2 Create an audit checklist

    3.3 Select a checklist to apply to the current audit

    3.4 View and update the checklist

4.0 Reporting an audit

5.0 Recording audit nonconformances

6.0 Preparing an audit report

7.0 Tracking audits (view by actual dates of audit, by dates and summary, by auditors)

8.0 Analyzing audit performance

    8.1 Areas of the standard (analysis to ensure each area of the standard has been audited in all appropriate departments)

    8.2 Documents (analysis to ensure each controlled document associated with each department has been audited and the effectiveness of those audits)

    8.3 Audits (analysis of the number of times each area of standard, department, document has been audited)

    8.4 Auditors (analysis of the effectiveness of each auditor)

Figure 11.7 The steps to be taken in conducting an audit (Q-Pulse)

The procedure for audit (Figure 11.3) makes reference to the Q-Pulse Manual and Figure 11.7 shows the steps that need to be taken in Q-Pulse in order to conduct an audit and these steps are common to any type of audit. Examples of forms on which the different audits are recorded are shown in Figures 11.11 and 11.12 and Figure 11.19 shows a form for registering and managing nonconformities.

The audit forms and the registration of nonconformities form between them, should include the following information, name(s) of the auditor(s), date of audit, a reference number, details of activities, areas or items audited, any nonconformities or deficiencies found, recommendations and timescales for corrective action/preventive action, responsibilities, and the name and signature of the individual confirming completion of corrective/preventive action.

ASSESSMENT OF USER SATISFACTION AND COMPLAINTS (INCLUDING CLINICAL AUDIT)

'Ideal Standard' clause 8.21 Assessment of user satisfaction and complaints(including clinical audit)
This section deals with the two issues that relate to the user, user satisfaction (including clinical audit) and users complaints.

ASSESSMENT OF USER SATISFACTION/CLINICAL AUDIT

The audits/assessment conducted under this heading fall into the category of co-operative audits. In certain situations it is valuable for a laboratory to conduct a 'user satisfaction survey', and in the case of the user as the patient, these may be a useful exercise. Regular contact with the user, as the clinician, at clinico-pathological conferences, at regular meetings between groups of surgeons and histopathologists or through the consultation process is a further method of assessing user satisfaction. Whatever the method it is important, both for purposes of accreditation and for continuing professional development programmes, that where possible records are kept of such activities.

However, more fundamental value is to be gained by assessing the clinical effectiveness (and efficiency) of the laboratory. This can either be done by using 'surrogate markers' to assess the effectiveness of the laboratory or by participation in the clinical audit/clinical effectiveness activities of the hospital. A recent paper (see Appendix 2, Further reading) argues that efficiency and effectiveness are linked, and suggests a practical approach by putting forward a ten point list of markers to stimulate activity. The approach includes, laboratory incident reporting, audit of quality of comments on clinical reports (from the view point of 'added value'), identification of undiagnosed conditions and appropriateness of laboratory assay repertoire. At St Elsewhere's, as well as a formal documentation of laboratory incidents, a proactive approach is taken using horizontal audits of say, quality of clinical data provided by the user. Appendix 2, Further reading, cites a book entitled, 'Laboratory-Related Measures of Patient Outcomes:an income' that is an important contribution to a complex area.

Clinical or medical audit may be thought of as a recent innovation, but Florence Nightingale in a methodical assessment of the standards of medical care in Army hospitals in the Crimea, showed that 'the key determinant of regimental mortality was distance from hospital. The least fortunate regiments were those with good access to hospital beds, because deaths depended less on casualties in battle than on acquiring an infection in hospital', an excellent example of clinical audit which has its echoes in the modern day problems with Methicillin resistant *Staphylococcus aureus*.

It is salutary to realise that as long ago as 1919, 'The Minimum Standard' promulgated by the American College of Surgeons of North America, included in Section 4 a description of doctors organizing themselves as a professional body and conducting medical audit on a regular basis (Figure 11.8).

In that the staff initiate and, with the approval of the governing board of the hospital, adopt rules, regulations and policies governing the professional work of the hospital; that these rules, regulations, and policies specifically provide:

(a) That staff meetings be held at least once each month. (In large hospitals the departments may chose to meet separately).

(b) That the staff review and analyze at regular intervals their clinical experience in the various departments of the hospital, such as medicine, surgery, obstetrics, and the other specialities; the clinical records of patients, free and pay, to be the basis for such review and analyses.

Figure 11.8 Section 4 of The Minimum Standard

John Gabbay defined clinical audit as '...colleagues reflecting on their work systematically, critically and openly, to enable them to agree how to do it better and check improvements occur'. The key issues are a systematic and critical approach, the involvement of all appropriate staff, and focus on patient care. Clinical audit is essentially a form of quality audit intended to lead to the maintenance and/or improvement in clinical effectiveness. It has a lot in common with the internal audit of examination processes but with its primary focus on patient outcome rather than on pre-examination, examination and post-examination processes themselves. The first step is the identification of an issue or topic for audit, such as,

- Is the correct action taken when a patient is found to have a low sodium or a high potassium?

- How many patients with high TSH values have regular monitoring following treatment?

- Does the laboratory follow up a high mean cell volume with appropriate tests?

The next step is to determine the purpose and nature of the service provided and perform a literature search to see if there is any previous work on the topic. Then follows the negotiation of an agreed procedure and determination of the objective criteria against which practice can be measured. After monitoring practice, an evaluation takes place. If the criteria have not been met, options for change have to be considered and a plan made to implement the change. If necessary the procedure is then re-negotiated and the cycle repeated. Implementation of change is crucial if improvements in healthcare outcome are to be effected. To be effective, implementation of change should come about through education rather than by management dictate.

ASSESSMENT OF USERS COMPLAINTS
At St Elsewhere's all complaints, verbal or written, are recorded on a user complaint form [QF-GEN-UserCpt] shown in Figure 11.9. All complaints are registered as nonconformities on Q-Pulse by the Quality Manager. They are dealt with in the first instance by the Head of Department, or depending on the seriousness of the issue, by the Director of Pathology. It is the policy at St Elsewhere's that complaints made by members of the laboratory staff against users (e.g. unreasonable requests for examinations outside the routine day or verbal abuse) are also registered as complaints, hence the 'for or against' item on the form. The maxim, that 'the customer is always right' may be worth remembering, (even though they may be wrong!), but equally within the laboratory a 'no blame approach' can be important in establishing the truth of any situation.

STAFF SUGGESTIONS
In Chapter 3, the principles of management were discussed and the involvement of people stressed. At St Elsewhere's, managing quality is seen very much as a bottom up process, in which maximum involvement of staff is encouraged. One way of facilitating this is through staff suggestions as to any improvements that

can be made. These range from better lighting outside the laboratory at night, to changing the plastic containers used for 24 hour urine collections. A 'staff suggestion' form [QF-GEN-StafSug] is used, which is identical to the user complaint form shown in Figure 11.9 except that the word 'complaint' is replaced by 'suggestion'. Suggestions are recorded in Q-pulse as nonconformities.

USER COMPLAINTS FORM

RECORD FILENAME	QF-GEN-UserCpt # NC-01-00031

1 Nonconformity no.	2 Complainant	3 Person dealing with the complaint
NC-01-00031	Dr H R Tetchley, Consultant Physician	Dr Alfred Johnson, Head of Biochemistry

4 Date of complaint	5 Date closed	6 Department
03 April 2001	12 April 2001	Biochemistry

7 Complaint (for or against)	By the user #	Against a user #

8 Nature of the complaint

A letter attached details the complaint. The turnaround time for Prolactin assays over the last month has been getting worse and I don't think the results are correct'. Details of three patients attached.

9 Results of investigation of the complaint

The internal quality control results and external quality assessment results were checked for the period when the patients results were analyzed and found to be within the standard set. However it was noted that the dates written on the request form were all one week earlier than the date the sample was received in the laboratory. It was determined that the courier service from the private hospital concerned had left the samples in the van for four days before delivery.

10 Corrective or preventative action taken

a)   a letter was sent to Dr Tetchley giving details of the investigation of the complaint and indicating that preventative action b) and c) had been taken, and thanking him for drawing the laboratory's attention to the problem (copy attached)

b)   letter sent to CEO of the private hospital regarding the performance of the courier service (copy attached)

c)   reception staff were asked to draw to the attention of the Head of Department IMMEDIATELY, any large discrepancies between date on request form and day of receipt

11 Person discharging the complaint	12 Signature of Head of department	13 Date
J Qualiman	Alfred Johnson	14April '02

Figure 11.9 Completed form for registering complaints [QF-GEN-UserCpt]

INTERNAL AUDIT OF THE QUALITY MANAGEMENT SYSTEM
'Ideal Standard' clause 8.2.2 Internal audit of the quality management system

At St Elsewhere's the horizontal audit is used and the objective is that all appropriate requirements of the 'Ideal Standard' are examined throughout the Pathology Laboratory in the course of a year. The main focus of audit in this area is on the proper functioning of all aspects of the quality management system such as document control, control of records/clinical material and the management of resources. These elements provide essential support to the examination processes. Audits in this area would seek to establish whether all procedures in use were up to date and being properly followed. For example, a simple check will confirm that all procedures being used are in date, but establishing that they are being properly followed requires evidence. This is found by examining the records created by completion of the appropriate forms.

INTERNAL AUDIT OF EXAMINATION PROCESSES
'Ideal Standard' clause 8.2.3 Internal audit of examination processes

At St Elsewhere's vertical and witness audits are used. The application of vertical audits to examination processes has two main purposes, firstly, the retrospective investigation of a nonconformity (see clause 8.4 of the 'Ideal Standard') discovered in the result of an examination that has already been authorized and issued and secondly, the proactive use of a vertical audit to ensure that the examination processes are being operated in compliance with procedures. In order for a prospective vertical audit to be of value it must investigate all the factors that ensure the proper conduct of the particular examination. These factors are illustrated in Figure 11.10.

The scope when a vertical audit is used to investigate a nonconformity depends on the nature of the nonconformity and may be satisfied by inspection of internal quality control results and external quality assessment scheme performance, or may lead to investigation of other issues relating to pre-examination processes such as specimen collection, handling, transportation and reception. The investigation of the user complaint illustrated in Figure 11.9, used a vertical audit approach to determine the factors that caused the complaint. An example of the structure of the form used at St Elsewhere's to conduct prospective vertical audits is shown in Figure 11.11.

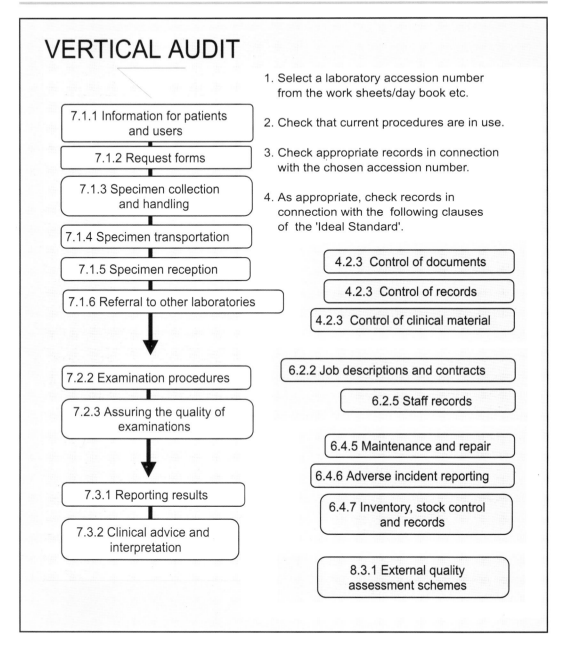

VERTICAL AUDIT

1. Select a laboratory accession number from the work sheets/day book etc.

2. Check that current procedures are in use.

3. Check appropriate records in connection with the chosen accession number.

4. As appropriate, check records in connection with the following clauses of the 'Ideal Standard'.

7.1.1 Information for patients and users

7.1.2 Request forms

7.1.3 Specimen collection and handling

7.1.4 Specimen transportation

7.1.5 Specimen reception

7.1.6 Referral to other laboratories

4.2.3 Control of documents

4.2.3 Control of records

4.2.3 Control of clinical material

7.2.2 Examination procedures

7.2.3 Assuring the quality of examinations

6.2.2 Job descriptions and contracts

6.2.5 Staff records

6.4.5 Maintenance and repair

6.4.6 Adverse incident reporting

6.4.7 Inventory, stock control and records

7.3.1 Reporting results

7.3.2 Clinical advice and interpretation

8.3.1 External quality assessment schemes

Figure 11.10 Vertical audit of examination processes

VERTICAL AUDIT FORM			
RECORD FILENAME		*QF-GEN-VertAud # VA-03-00034*	

1 Audit No.	2 Audit title	3 Auditor(s)
VA-01-00034	*Vertical audit*	*Jane Rubin/John Lipton*

4 Date opened (date performed)	5 Date closed (date all NC's closed)	6 Department
03 March 2001		*Biochemistry*

7 Area of standard	8 Procedure/examination involved
7 Examination processes	*LP-BIO-BHMMan / liver profile*

9 Audit findings

Audit area	Records checked	Observations	NC no.
7.1.1 Information for users and patients	*Users handbook*	*Information available*	*-*
7.1.2 Request form	*Request form Accession no. BC 006521*	*Date of request, 09Jan'01 Blood on the request form*	*NC-01-00043*
7.1.3 Specimen collection and handling	*Request form Accession no. BC 006521*	*Date of collection, 10Jan'01 Blood on specimen container*	*NC-01-00043*
7.1.4 Specimen transportation	*Courier service*	*No comments*	*-*

10 Person closing the audit	11 Signature of Head of department/section	12 Date

Figure 11.11 The vertical audit form (examination processes) [QF-GEN-VertAud]

It resulted in the discovery of one nonconformity regarding blood on the request form and specimen container. This nonconformity is recorded in the right hand column of section 9 as nonconformity number (NC no), NC-01-00001 where NC=Nonconformity, -01=2001, -00043= nonconformity number 43.

At St Elsewhere's the witness audit is used to check that an individual has a thorough understanding of the work they are undertaking and the training programme is an essential prerequisite to a member of staff being certified as competent to perform a particular procedure (see Figure 6.17 showing a partially completed training record). An example of a witness audit form is shown in Figure 11.12. It resulted in the discovery of one nonconformity regarding the involvement of staff in the review of results from an EQAS, recorded in the right hand column of section 9 as nonconformity number (NC no), NC-01-00001 where NC=Nonconformity, -01=2001, -00001= nonconformity number one.

WITNESS AUDIT FORM

RECORD FILENAME	QF-GEN-WitnAud # WA-01-00001

1 Audit No.	2 Operator witnessed	3 Auditor/witness
WA-01-00001	Jane Rubin	John Lipton

4 Date opened (date performed)	5 Date closed (date all NC's closed)	6 Department
03 Jan 2001		Biochemistry

7 Area of standard	8 Procedure/examination involved
7 Examination processes	LP-BIO-HBA1c

9 Audit findings-compliance and understanding of the procedure

Item	Observations	NC no.
Content of procedure	good	-
Calibration	good	-
Reagents	good	-
Internal quality control	good	-
External quality assessment	Not involved in reviewing results	NC-01-00001

10 Person closing the audit	11 Signature of Head of department/section	12 Date

Figure 11.12 Witness audit form [QF-GEN-WitnAud]

EXTERNAL AUDIT
'Ideal Standard' clause 8.3 External audit

There are two main forms of external audit, firstly, the laboratory participating in appropriate external quality assessment schemes (EQAS) and secondly, external reports based upon assessment/inspections made by outside bodies.

EXTERNAL QUALITY ASSESSMENT SCHEMES
'Ideal Standard' clause 8.3.1 External quality assessment schemes
In pathology the terms 'internal quality control' and 'external quality assessment' (proficiency testing) are perhaps the most familiar, although in the past the term 'external quality control' was frequently used instead of external quality assessment. A useful definition of external quality assessment is given in Figure 11.13 and contrasting this with the definition of internal quality control from the same source, (Figure 10.18), serves to reinforce their distinctly different roles in assuring the quality of examinations.

External quality assessment.....

'... refers to a system of objectively checking laboratory results by means of an external agency. The checking is necessarily retrospective, and the comparison of a given laboratory's performance on a certain day with that of other laboratories cannot be notified to the laboratory until some time later. This comparison will not therefore have any influence on the tested laboratory's output on the day of the test. The main object of EQA is not to bring about day to day consistency but to establish between-laboratory comparability'

WHO External Assessment of Health Laboratories (1981)

Figure 11.13 Definition of external quality assessment

The essential difference between quality control and quality assessment is the time frame in which remedial action can be taken. For example, if a batch of examinations is performed and the results on quality control samples are outside agreed limits, then the results on patient samples can be withheld and the batch repeated. In other words 'the stable door can be closed before the horse has bolted'. On the other hand, if the results on external quality assessment samples are found to be outside acceptable limits then all that can be done is to instigate a retrospective investigation of that particular examination. 'Many horses may have bolted in the meantime!'. In this text quality control is used in an operational sense and results in 'immediate feedback control'.

However, the existence of quality assessment schemes has been one of the key factors in the improvement of pathology examinations. R J Maxwell, in his article on quality assessment in health, said 'There are undoubtedly some outstanding examples of quality assessment activities in health services in Britain such as the confidential enquiry into maternal deaths, or the national quality control scheme in clinical chemistry' (as it was then called). In the same article he describes the scheme with commendable brevity. 'The scheme began in 1969. Every two weeks a portion of material is sent to all participating laboratories for analysis. They return their results of several commonly performed tests, and the data from all laboratories are compared. For each of the principal laboratory methods in use, the mean value, standard deviation, and variance index are calculated, thus each laboratory can compare its results to others while confidentiality is respected. Those who administer the scheme have been able to show progressive reduction in variance index, thus showing improvement in the consistency of results obtained by different laboratories'.

There are now an amazing diversity of schemes covering all disciplines of pathology. In many countries they were originally nurtured in the protective environment of the national healthcare schemes or in centres of academic excellence, but increasingly excellent schemes have become available from commercial sources for the more routine assays. However, the practical problems of setting up, for example, the UK scheme for breast screening pathology with its 300 UK participants, are of a magnitude greater than those of a general clinical chemistry scheme with 600 participants. Even so, obtaining material which is commutable with human samples still poses problems in clinical chemistry.

The process of a laboratory participating in EQAS involvement is shown in Figure 11.14.

A procedure for the management of participation in EQAS's is one the most important in the laboratory. At St Elsewhere's each department has its own procedure [QP-XXX-EQAMan], but they follow an identical structure which is shown in Figure 11.15.

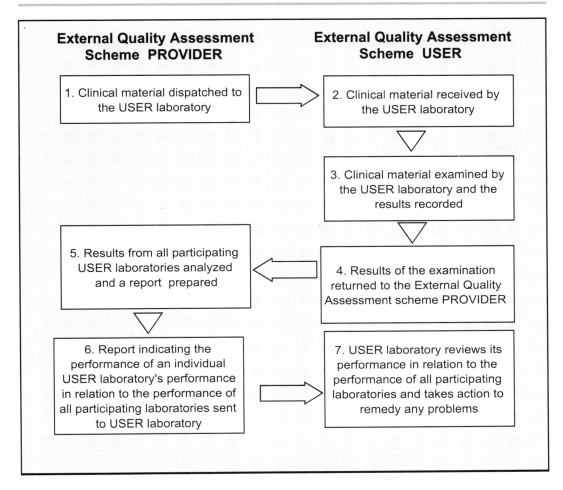

Figure 11.14 External quality assessment schemes-process

0 INTRODUCTION 0.1 Purpose and scope 0.2 Responsibility 0.3 References 0.4 Definitions 0.5 Documentation	**5 RECEIPT AND REVIEW OF SCHEME REPORTS**
1 RECEIPT AND LOGGING OF SAMPLES	**6 ACTION IN RESPONSE TO PROBLEMS**
2 ACCESSION OF SAMPLES	**7 REVIEW OF SCHEME PARTICIPATION**
3 SAMPLE ANALYSIS	**8 RECEIPT AND REVIEW OF SCHEME ANNUAL REPORTS**
4 RESULT REPORTING	**9 RECORDS**

Figure 11.15 Contents for the procedure for management of participation in external quality assessment schemes [QP-XXX-EQAMan]

For participation to be effective, two issues are crucial, firstly, proper records must be kept of the results obtained in the laboratory, (of the nonconformities (aberrant results) reported and the corrective/preventive actions which result), and secondly, the findings must be discussed with all the staff involved in the particular examinations. A form designed to follow the process (Figure 11.14) is shown in Figure 11.16. At the present time at St Elsewhere's, the nonconformities found are not entered into Q-Pulse, but action to be taken is closely monitored at department quality meetings and any outstanding serious problems reported to the Quality and Accreditation Committee of the laboratory.

In many schemes there are advantages of participation that go beyond the ability to compare the performance of one's own laboratory against the overall performance of other laboratories. Schemes that deal with quantitative assays will subdivide the participants into method groups or instrumentation groups, and this enables the participant to judge whether they are 'running with the tide' or whether they stand in splendid isolation and still use Folin and Wu's technique for blood sugar assays! This data also informs the laboratory of trends in different methods of measurement, for example, the change from gas chromatographic techniques to fluorescent polarisation or enzyme mediated immunoassays in therapeutic drug monitoring.

EQA MANAGEMENT FORM

RECORD FILENAME	

1 Department	2 Section

3 Supervisor's name	4 Scheme name

5 Sample identification(s)	6 Date sample received*

7 Date results returned (copy attached)	8 Date report received (copy attached)

9 Report discussed with (enter name)	10 Date report discussed

11 Action to be taken

Observations	Action to be taken and by who	Target date for completion	Date nonconformity discharged

* Please note here if discrepancy between date received and expected date of receipt			

Figure 11.16 Form for recording participation in external quality assessment schemes [QF-XXX-EQAMan]

A further important aspect of EQAS is their use in the assessment of clinical interpretation. An example is the UK NEQAS Clinical Chemistry scheme for 'Assessment of Clinical Interpretation'. In this web-based scheme, a brief case history and/or laboratory results are provided and 'value-added comments' invited. When the case is 'closed' the comments of the participants (anonymised) are sent to a panel of expert assessors who give a mark, from +2 (highly appropriate) to -2 (highly inappropriate) to each comment. This results in an average mark for each participant's individual comment, and this is included in a personalised report for each participant. The individualised report is posted on the web, and contains the case pathophysiology, background education and expert opinion, plus examples of selected comments which illustrate good and not so good practice. A positive score for a participant indicates that they are 'adding value' to a set of results and vice versa. This approach brings into play not only the ability of a laboratory to produce accurate results, but also confirms that they are being correctly interpreted in the context of the clinical situation.

RELATIONSHIP TO ACCREDITATION
Participation in recognised or approved quality assessment or proficiency testing schemes is an essential requirement for accreditation and in many countries the laboratory's performance in the schemes has not only become an integral part of the accreditation process, but the determinant of whether the laboratory can continue to operate or get reimbursed for their work. Some accreditation bodies develop and operate their own EQASs and some depend upon external agencies to provide schemes.

ACCREDITATION OF QUALITY ASSESSMENT SCHEMES
When an accreditation body makes a statement to the effect that laboratories must participate in approved external assessment schemes, it raises the issue of what is to be considered as an approved scheme. The ILAC publication, ILAC-G13-2000: 'Guidelines for the requirements for the competence of providers of proficiency testing schemes' is 'directed to providers of proficiency schemes who wish, on a voluntary basis, to demonstrate their competence, for the purpose of accreditation or other recognition, by formal compliance with a set of internationally acceptable requirements for the planning and implementation of proficiency testing schemes'.

It cross references with ISO Guide-1 1997 'Proficiency testing by interlaboratory comparisons – Part 1: Development and operation of proficiency testing schemes' and ISO Guide 43-2: 1997 'Proficiency testing by interlaboratory comparisons – Part 2: Selection and use of proficiency testing schemes by laboratory accreditation bodies', the requirements of which it regards as 'a sound basis' for the selection of schemes by laboratories and their acceptance during laboratory assessment. In Australia and the UK standards have been promulgated by national accrediting bodies for acceptance of schemes specifically for medical laboratories (see Appendix 2, Further reading). The CPA(UK)Ltd standards which are used as a basis for accreditation of EQASs in the UK are based upon and cross referenced to the ILAC and ISO standards.

EXTERNAL REVIEWS

'Ideal Standard' clause 8.3.2 External reviews

In relation to accreditation, the most immediately relevant reports are those that come from the accreditation bodies and detail any noncompliances with the standards. The noncompliances have to be rectified within a specified time frame in order for accreditation status to be maintained. During the initial development of voluntary accreditation schemes, states of partial or conditional accreditation are sometimes recognised. However, as the schemes mature it is important from the point of view of the user that a clear statement is made to signify that either a laboratory is accredited, or not. To do otherwise will eventually lead to a lack of credibility in the process of assessment and the accreditation body.

The other important source of external review comes from inspections sometimes conducted as a result of national regulations (e.g. health and safety, radiological protection and fire inspections) or by governmental audit bodies, that can relate to financial as well as service issues.

NONCONFORMING EXAMINATIONS

'Ideal Standard' clause 8.4 Nonconforming examinations

In ISO 9001:2000, ISO 17025:1999 and ISO 15189:2002 the relevant clauses are respectively 8.3, 4.9 and 4.9 (see Appendix 1) and all contain the word 'control' in the title of the clause. In ISO 9001:2000 the clause is concerned with ensuring that a 'product that does not conform to product requirements is identified and controlled to prevent its unintended use or delivery'. Later in the clause however, it comments on the situation where the 'nonconforming product is detected after delivery or use' and requires that 'the organization shall take action appropriate to the effects, or potential effects of the nonconformity'. This situation is mirrored in the comparable clauses of ISO 17025:1999 and ISO 15189:2002. From the standpoint of a medical laboratory, the use of the word 'control' in relation to the first activity, would be regarded as the function of internal quality control, preventing nonconforming results being issued, whereas the second activity would be seen as remedial action or as has been said earlier, action 'after the horse has bolted'! Both activities are extremely important and at St Elsewhere's the internal quality control activity is dealt with in the appropriate examination procedures (LP-) and the second activity in the procedure for management of evaluation and continual improvement [QP-GEN-Eval&CI] and in some departments in reporting procedures [LP-XXX-Report].

IMPROVEMENT

'Ideal Standard' clause 8.5 Improvement

In ISO 9001:2000, clause 8.5 is simply titled *'Improvement'* and embraces the three aspects of continual improvement, corrective action and preventive action. It can be seen from Figure 11.1 (and in Appendix 1), that the clauses of the 'Ideal Standard' follow this arrangement. In ISO 17025:1999 there is no clause entitled 'continual improvement' although the concept is implicit in much of the Standard. All three aspects of improvement have separate clauses in ISO 15189:2002. ISO 9001:2000 describes the content of the rest of this chapter, in the requirement that, 'the organization shall continually improve the effectiveness of the quality management system, through the use of its quality policy, quality objectives, audit results, analysis of data, corrective and preventive actions and management review'.

CONTINUAL IMPROVEMENT
'Ideal Standard' clause 8.5.1 Continual improvement
A representation of this activity is shown in Fig 11.17, in what the author has termed 'cycles of continual improvement'. The intention of the diagram is to represent at the centre, the management review as the core focus of all continual improvement activity. The cycles around the central circle represent individual circles of continual improvement focused on specific topics, for example, with 6.2 Personnel, the activity is the annual joint review of staff (Figure 6.11), with 8.2.3 Internal audit of examination processes, the vertical audit of examinations (Figure 11.11) and with 6.4 Equipment and diagnostic systems, the procurement of IVDs (Figure 8.6).

An important question to answer at this point is when and how often should these activities take place. These cycles of continual improvement carry on throughout the year and most of the nonconformities produced have to be resolved in a reasonably short time span for the process to be effective. However, during the course of a year, issues that require the formal setting of new objectives and detailed planning will be identified and these properly go forward as items for consideration at the (annual) management review. If the results from an EQAS indicate a problem with an examination, it is no good waiting until the management review for its resolution, whereas the requirement for new service provision may have to wait for the capital purchase of the appropriate IVD or the recruitment of new staff.

At St Elsewhere's Pathology Laboratory (which serves a resident population of 560,000 and has commensurate resources), the objective has been set that the laboratory will carry out two comprehensive health and safety audits (plus four on special topics), and internal (horizontal) audits that cover all aspects of the QMS during the course of a year. Additionally each department will undertake four internal (vertical) audits of examination processes in the year. The staff will have one joint review per year and staff will have witness audits if they are in training or new procedures are introduced. The vertical audits, if done thoroughly, have been found to be an extremely valuable exercise. As many as 95% of the staff take part in these activities each year and this includes the cleaning lady who has a fierce eye for unwarranted untidiness.

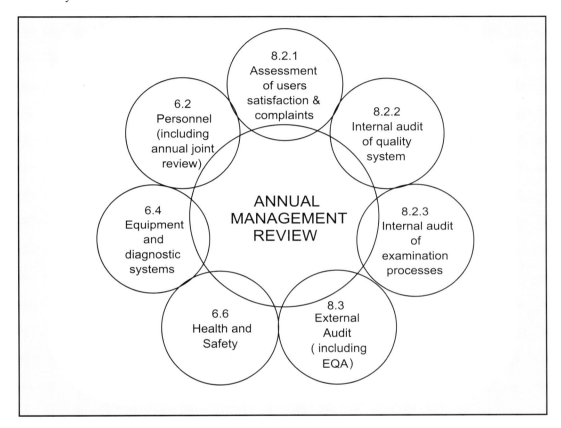

Figure 11.17 Cycles of continual improvement

NONCONFORMITY

The nonconformities that are thrown up during the day to day activities of quality management are the 'grist to the mill' (defined in common English usage as 'anything that can be turned to profit or advantage') of continual improvement, or the cogs in the cycles of continual improvement. Nonconformities arise from a number of different routes and these are illustrated in relation to clauses of the 'Ideal Standard' in Figure 11.18.

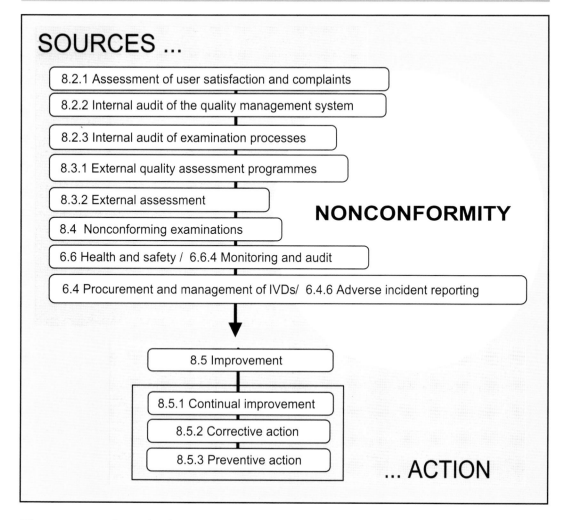

SOURCES ...

8.2.1 Assessment of user satisfaction and complaints

8.2.2 Internal audit of the quality management system

8.2.3 Internal audit of examination processes

8.3.1 External quality assessment programmes

8.3.2 External assessment

8.4 Nonconforming examinations

6.6 Health and safety / 6.6.4 Monitoring and audit

6.4 Procurement and management of IVDs/ 6.4.6 Adverse incident reporting

NONCONFORMITY

8.5 Improvement

8.5.1 Continual improvement

8.5.2 Corrective action

8.5.3 Preventive action

... ACTION

Figure 11.18 The 'Ideal Standard' – Sources and action in relation to nonconformity

When a nonconformity is identified, by whatever means, it must be recorded in order that its progress through corrective or preventive action can be followed leading to its eventual discharge. The form that has been used at St Elsewhere's for this purpose is shown in Figure 11.19. The example shown recorded a nonconformity found in a horizontal audit of all staff in the laboratory on an area of the 'Ideal Standard' that requires that staff complete an induction programme.

NONCONFORMITY FORM

RECORD FILENAME	*QF-GEN-NonConf# NC-02-00078*

1 Nonconformity No.	2 Source	3 Responsibility
NC-02-00078	*Horizontal audit*	*John Lipton*

4 Date opened	5 Date closed	6 Department
03 April 2000		*Biochemistry*

7 Area of standard	8 Procedure/examination involved
6.2.3 Induction and orientation	

9 Nonconformity

One member of staff with incomplete induction /health and safety training incomplete

10 Corrective or preventive action taken

11 Person discharging the nonconformity	12 Signature of Head of Department	13 Date

Figure 11.19 Partially completed form for recording nonconformities [QF-GEN-NonConf]

CORRECTIVE ACTION / PREVENTIVE ACTION

'Ideal Standard' clauses 8.5.2 Corrective action and 8.5.3 Preventive action

Definitions of corrective and preventive action are shown in Figure 11.2 and examples have been provided to illustrate the definitions. In relation to both corrective and preventive action, ISO 9001:2000 requires a documented procedure that defines the requirements for reviewing the nonconformities identified, determining their causes, evaluating, determining and implementing a course of action, and recording and subsequently reviewing the action taken. At St Elsewhere's this is a section of the procedure for the management of evaluation and continual improvement, (Figure 11.3).

MANAGEMENT REVIEW
'Ideal Standard' clause 5.3.7 Management review

ISO 9001:2000, ISO 17025:1999 and ISO 15189:2002 all have clauses entitled *'management review(s)'*, respectively 5.6, 4.14 and 4.15. In ISO 9001:2000, the responsibility for its conduct is defined as being with 'top management', in ISO 17025:1999, with 'the laboratory's executive management' and in ISO 15189:2002 with 'laboratory management'. The time interval for this activity is not defined in ISO 9001:2000, but notes in the other standards suggest that 'a typical period for conducting a management review is once every twelve months'. It is important that the review should be seen as having inputs and outputs and these are defined in general terms in ISO 9001:2000. The CPA(UK)Ltd, Standard A11 'Management review' has specific information regarding required inputs and Figure 11.20 is based on these requirements.

The **management review** shall include:

a) reports from managerial and supervisory personnel
b) assessment of user satisfaction and complaints
c) internal audit of quality management system
d) internal audit of examination processes
e) external quality assessment reports
f) reports of assessments by outside bodies
g) status of preventative, corrective and improvements actions
h) major changes in organization and management, resource (including staff) or process

based upon the CPA(UK)Ltd, Standard A11 Management review

Figure 11.20 Inputs to the management review

ISO 9001:2000, describes the output from the management review as including 'any decisions and actions related to a) improvement of the effectiveness of the QMS and its processes, b) improvement of the product related to customer requirements, and c) resource needs'.

At St Elsewhere's the management review is conducted on an annual basis and is integrated into the business planning cycle of the Trust. A special one day meeting of the Pathology Management Board is held in September, (the financial year commences in April), and follows an agenda as shown in Figure 11.21. All the reports which serve as inputs to the review are prepared according to a proforma and circulated one month in advance of the meeting.

INPUTS

Reports from Heads of department

Report from the Quality Manager

Report from Health and Safety sub-committee

Report from the Business manager

Agenda - Annual management review

1. Present
2. Apologies for absence
3. Reports from Heads of Departments
   - Performance in EQA schemes
   - Clinical audits/clinical governance
   - New developments
4. Report from the Quality Manager
   - Customer complaints
   - Internal audit
   - External reports
5. Report from the Health and Safety Officer
6. Report from the Business Manager
   - Financial statement
   - IVD requests
   - New building developments
   - Staff requirements
7. Summary from the Director of Pathology
8. Draft annual management review
9. Acceptance of review for publication

Report of the annual management review

Contents
Executive summary
1 The past year...successes and failures
2 Needs and requirements of users
3 Resource management
   - personnel
   - premises
   - IVD procurement
4 Health and safety
5 Quality management (including clinical audit)
6 Financial requirements - capital and revenue
7 Future key objectives and priorities

OUTPUTS

Figure 11.21 Conduct of the annual management review

The responsibility for bringing together all the required information in a timely manner lies with the Quality Manager, who also works with the Director of

Pathology in advance of the review meeting to prepare a draft report of the review. The draft report is circulated in advance of the meeting and representatives of all departments must be present. The meeting is held off-site and items 1-5 are dealt with from 9.00-13.00 hr, and items 6-7 from 14.00-19.00 hr followed by an informal buffet supper. This day is the single most important day in the calender of the Pathology Laboratory and sets the objectives for the following year. These objectives are translated into objectives for individual departments, that in turn feed into the staff joint reviews that take place in January-March of the following year and underpin the continuing provision of a quality service that aims to meet the needs and requirements of the user.

Finally, the ideas that are put forward in this book and illustrated by life in the Pathology Laboratory of St Elsewhere's Hospital are based on the author's experience of a number of very different types of laboratories. If what is contained in this book contributes in any small way to improving the quality of the already excellent service provided by so many medical laboratories throughout the world, the staff at St Elsewhere's will regard their effort as having been well worthwhile.

Appendix 1

Standards cross-reference table

In the table below, clauses of the 'Ideal Standard' are cross referenced as far as is practicable with the following standards:

- ISO 9001:2000 Quality management systems – Requirements

- ISO/IEC 17025:1999 General requirements for the competence of testing and calibration laboratories

- ISO/IEC 15189:2002 Medical laboratories – Particular requirements for quality and competence

- CPA(UK)Ltd Standards for the Medical Laboratory.

In order to fully appreciate the relationship between the different standards it is necessary to have the full text.

'Ideal Standard'	ISO 9001:2000	ISO 17025:1999	ISO 1589:2002	CPA(UK)Ltd
4 Quality management system	**4 Quality management system**	**4.2 Quality system**	**4.2 Quality management system**	**A4 Quality management system**
4.1 General requirements	4.1 General requirements	4.2 Quality system	4.2 Quality management system	A4 Quality management system
4.2 Documentation requirements	4.2 Documentation requirements	4.2 Quality system	4.2 Quality management system	A4 Quality management system
4.2.1 General	4.2.1 General	*(as above)*	*(as above)*	*(as above)*
4.2.2 Quality manual	4.2.2 Quality manual	*(as above)*	*(as above)*	A6 Quality manual
4.2.3 Control of documents	4.2.3 Control of documents	4.3 Document control	4.3 Document control	A8 Document control
4.2.4 Control of records	4.2.4 Control of records	4.12 Control of records	4.13 Quality and technical records	A9 Control of process & quality records
4.2.5 Control of clinical material	*Not applicable*	-	-	A10 Control of clinical material
5 Organization & management responsibility	**5 Management responsibility**	**4 Management requirements**	**4 Management requirements**	**A1 Organisation and management**
5.1 General management	*Not applicable*	4.1 Organisation	4.1 Organisation and management	A1 Organisation and management
5.2 Organisation	*Not applicable*	4.1 Organisation	4.1 Organisation and management	A1 Organisation and management
5.3 Management responsibility	5 Management responsibility	4.1 Organisation	4.1 Organisation and management	B1 Professional direction
5.3.1 Management commitment	5.1 Management commitment	4.2 Quality system	4.2 Quality management system	-
5.3.2 Needs and requirements of the users	5.2 Customer focus	4.4 Review of requests, tenders and contacts	4.4 Review of contracts	A2 Needs and requirements of users
5.3.3 Quality policy	5.3 Quality policy	4.2 Quality system	4.2 Quality management system	A3 Quality policy
5.3.4 Quality objectives and plans	5.4 Planning	*(as above)*	*(as above)*	A5 Quality objectives and plans
5.3.5 Responsibility, authority and communication	5.5 Responsibility, authority and communication	*(as above)*	*(as above)*	A1 Organisation and management
5.3.6 Quality manager	5.5.2 Management representative	*(as above)*	*(as above)*	A7 Quality manager
5.3.7 Management review	5.6 Management review	4.14 Management review	4.15 Management review	A11 Management review

'Ideal Standard'	ISO 9001:2000	ISO 17025:1999	ISO 1589:2002	CPA(UK)Ltd
6 Resource management	**6 Resource management**	**5 Technical requirements**	**5 Technical requirements**	**Sections B, C & D**
6.1 Provision of resources	6.1 Provision of resources	5.1 General		Sections B, C and D
6.2 Personnel	6.2 Human resources	5.2 Personnel	5.1 Personnel	Section B
6.2.1 General requirements	6.2.1 General	5.2 Personnel	5.1 Personnel	B1 Professional direction B2 Staffing B3 Personnel management
6.2.2 Job descriptions and contracts		*(as above)*	*(as above)*	B5 Job descriptions and contracts
6.2.3 Induction and orientation		*(as above)*	*(as above)*	B4 Staff orientation and induction
6.2.4 Annual joint review		*(as above)*	*(as above)*	B7 Staff annual joint review
6.2.5 Staff records	6.2.2 Competence, awareness and training	*(as above)*	*(as above)*	B6 Staff records
6.2.6 Competence, awareness and training	6.2.2 Competence, awareness and training	*(as above)*	*(as above)*	B9 Staff training and education
6.2.7 Meetings and communication				B8 Staff meetings
6.3 Premises	6.3 Infrastructure	5.3 Accommodation and environmental conditions	5.2 Accommodation and environmental conditions	Section C
6.3.1 General requirements				C1 Premises and environment
6.3.2 Laboratory and office facilities				C1 Premises and environment
6.3.3 Staff facilities				C2 Facilities for staff
6.3.4 Patient facilities				C3 Facilities for patients
6.3.5 Storage				C4 Facilities for storage

'Ideal Standard'	ISO 9001:2000	ISO 17025:1999	ISO 1589:2002	CPA(UK)Ltd
6 Resource management	**6 Resource management**	**5 Technical requirements**	**5 Technical requirements**	**Sections B, C & D**
6.4 Equipment & diagnostic systems	6.3 Infrastructure 7.4 Purchasing	5.5 Equipment	5.3 Laboratory equipment	Section D
6.4.1 Procurement and management	7.4.1 Purchasing process	4.6 Purchasing services and supplies	4.6 External services and supplies	D1 Procurement and management of equipment
6.4.2 Instructions for use				
6.4.3 Training				
6.4.4 Acceptance testing, user verification and validation	7.4.3 Verification of purchased product			
6.4.5 Maintenance and repair				
6.4.6 Adverse incident reporting				
6.4.7 Inventory, stock control and records	7.4.4 Purchasing information			D3 Management of reagents, calibration and quality control materials
6.5 Management of data and information systems	6.3 Infrastructure 7.4 Purchasing	5.5 Equipment	Annex B Laboratory information systems	D2 Management of data and information
6.5.1 General requirements				
6.5.2 Validation				
6.5.3 Security				
6.5.4 Maintenance and disaster recovery				
6.5.5 Archiving and retrieval				
6.5.6 Documentation				

'Ideal Standard'	ISO 9001:2000	ISO 17025:1999	ISO 1589:2002	CPA(UK)Ltd
6 Resource management	**6 Resource management**	**5 Technical requirements**	**5 Technical requirements**	**Sections B, C & D**
6.6 Health and safety	6.4 Work environment	5.3 Accommodation & environmental conditions	5.2 Accommodation & environmental conditions	C5 Health and safety
6.6.1 General requirements				
6.6.2 Hazards and risk assessment				
6.6.3 Accident and incident reporting				
6.6.4 Monitoring and audit				
6.6.5 Information, education and training				
6.6.6 Environmental effect				
7 Examination processes	**7 Product realization**	**5 Technical requirements**	**5 Technical requirements**	**Sections E, F & G**
7.1 Pre-examination process			5.4 Pre-examination procedures	Section E
7.1.1 Information for patients and users	7.2 Customer related processes 7.2.3 Customer communication	4.7 Service to the client	4.7 Advisory services	E1 Information for patients and users
7.1.2 Request form			5.5 Examination procedures	E2 Request form
7.1.3 Specimen collection and handling	7.5.5 Preservation of product	5.7 Sampling 5.8 Handling of test and calibration items	*(as above)*	E3 Specimen collection and handling
7.1.4 Specimen transportation	7.5.5 Preservation of product	*(as above)*	*(as above)*	E4 Specimen transportation
7.1.5 Specimen reception		*(as above)*	*(as above)*	E5 Specimen reception
7.1.6 Referral to other laboratories		4.5 Subcontracting of tests and calibrations	4.5 Examination by referral laboratories	E6 Referral to other laboratories

'Ideal Standard'	ISO 9001:2000	ISO 17025:1999	ISO 1589:2002	CPA(UK)Ltd
7 Examination processes	**7 Product realization**	**5 Technical requirements**	**5 Technical requirements**	**Sections E, F & G**
7.2 Examination process	7.5 Production and service provision		5.5 Examination procedures	Section F
7.2.1 Selection and validation of examination procedures	7.2.1 Determination of requirements related to the product 7.2.2 Review of requirements related to the product 7.5.2 Validation of processes for production and service provision 7.5.3 Identification and traceability	5.4 Test and calibration methods *and method validation* 5.6 Measurement traceability	5.5 Examination procedures	F1 Selection and validation of examination procedures
7.2.2 Examination procedures	7.1 Planning of product realization 7.3 Design and development	5.4 *Test and calibration methods* and method validation	5.5 Examination procedures	F2 Examination procedures
7.2.3 Assuring the quality of examinations	7.5.1 Control of production and service provision 7.6 Control of monitoring and measuring devices	5.9 Assuring the quality of test and calibration results	5.6 Assuring the quality of examinations	F3 Assuring the quality of examinations
7.3 Post-examination process	7.1 Planning of product realization 7.3 Design and development		5.7 Post-examination procedures	Section G
7.3.1 Reporting results		5.10 Reporting the results	5.8 Reporting of results 4.9 Identification and control of nonconformities	G1 Reporting results G2 The report G3 The telephoned report G4 The amended report
7.3.2 Clinical advice & interpretation	7.2.3 Customer communication	4.7 Service to the client	4.7 Advisory services	G5 Clinical advice and interpretation

'Ideal Standard'	ISO 9001:2000	ISO 17025:1999	ISO 1589:2002	CPA(UK)Ltd
8 Evaluation and continual improvement	**8 Measurement, analysis and improvement**	**4 Management requirements**	**4 Management requirements**	**Section H**
8.1 General	8.1 General			H1 Evaluation and improvement processes
8.2 Internal audit	8.2 Monitoring and measurement 8.4 Analysis of data			
8.2.1 Assessment of user satisfaction and complaint	8.2.1 Customer satisfaction	4.8 Complaints	4.8 Resolution of complaints	H2 Assessment of user satisfaction and complaint
8.2.2 Internal audit of the quality management system	8.2.2 Internal audit	4.13 Internal audits	4.14 Internal audits	H3 Internal audit of the quality management system
8.2.3 Internal audit of examination processes	8.2.3 Monitoring and measurement of processes	4.13 Internal audits 5.9 Assuring the quality or test and calibration results	4.14 Internal audits 5.6 Assuring the quality of examination processes	H4 Internal audit of examination processes
8.3 External audit				H5 External quality assessment
8.3.1 External quality assessment schemes	8.2.4 Monitoring and measurement of product	5.9 Assuring the quality of test and calibration results	5.6 Assuring the quality of examination processes	*(as above)*
8.3.2 External reviews				*(as above)*
8.4 Nonconforming examinations	8.3 Control of nonconforming product	4.9 Control of nonconforming testing and/or calibration work	4.9 Identification and control of nonconformities	
8.5 Improvement	8.5 Improvement			H6 Quality improvement
8.5.1 Continual improvement	8.5.1 Continual improvement		4.12 Continual improvement	*(as above)*
8.5.2 Corrective action	8.5.2 Corrective action	4.10 Corrective action	4.10 Corrective action	*(as above)*
8.5.3 Preventative action	8.5.3 Preventative action	4.11 Preventative action	4.11 Preventative action	*(as above)*

Appendix 2

Further reading

Attempts have been made, whereever possible to ensure that the material in Further Reading is available, if possible free of charge, from the World Wide Web. If the web site address is underlined the document can be downloaded free of charge, if the web site address is not underlined information can obtained as to how to obtain the document. The addresses given are to the home page and information can generally be found through a search engine on the site or through a document section.

Information regarding ISO and EN documents (which are not free of charge) can be found through national standards bodies a list of which can be found at www.iso.org. NCCLS documents can be ordered via the website, www.nccls.org. Documents marked with an asterisk in the author's opinion should be readily available as reference documents.

CHAPTER 1 – RECOGNITION OF MEDICAL LABORATORIES

Batjer JD. The College of American Pathologists laboratory accreditation programme. Clin Lab Haematol 1990; **12 (Suppl 1)**:135-8.

Burnett D. Understanding Accreditation in Laboratory Medicine, ACB Venture Publications, London, 1996 (www.acb.org.uk)

Pathology department accreditation in the United Kingdom: a synopsis. J Clin Pathol 1991; **44**: 798-802.

Principles of Clinical Laboratory Accreditation, A policy statement. IFCC and WASP, 1999 (www.ifcc.org).

CHAPTER 2 – THE CHANGING WORLD OF STANDARDS

*ISO 9001:2000 Quality management systems – Requirements.

*ISO/IEC 15189:2002 Medical Laboratories – Particular requirements for quality and competence.

*ISO/IEC 17025:1999 General requirements for the competence of testing and calibration laboratories.

Burnett D, Blair C. Standards for the medical laboratory – harmonisation and subsidiarity. Clin Chim Acta 2001; 309: 137-45.

Burnett D, Blair C, Haeney MR, Jeffcoate S,L, Scott KWM, Williams DL. Clinical pathology accreditation: standards for the medical laboratory. J Clin Pathol; 2002 **55:** 0-4.

Clinical Pathology Accreditation (UK)Ltd, Standards for the Medical Laboratory 2001 (www.cp-uk.co.uk).

College of American Pathologists, Standards for Laboratory Accreditation 1997 (www.cap.org).

Draft Standards for Pathology Laboratories, National Pathology Accreditation Advisory Council, Canberra, Australia, 2001 (www.health.gov.au/npaac).

International vocabulary of basic and general terms in metrology (VIM), issued by BIPM, IEC, IFCC, ISO, IUPAC, IUPAP and OIML.

ISO 14050:1998 Environment management – Vocabulary.

ISO Guide 2, General terms and their definitions concerning standardization and related activity.

ISO/IEC Directives, Part 1 Procedures for technical work, 4th edition, 2001.

ISO/IEC Directives, Part 2 Rules for the structure and drafting of International Standards4th edition, 2001

Jansen RTP, Blaton V, Burnett D, Huisman W, Queraltó JM, Zérah S, Allman B. Essential criteria for quality systems of medical laboratories. Eur J Clin Chem Clin Biochem 1997; **35:** 121-2 (www.uni-oldenberg.de/ec4/).

Jansen RTP, Blaton ,. Burnett D, Huisman W. Queraltó JM, Zérah S, Allman B. European Communities Confederation of Clinical Chemistry, Essential criteria for quality systems of medical laboratories. Eur J Clin Chem Clin Biochem 1997; **35:** 123-32 (www.uni-oldenberg.de/ec4/).

Jansen RTP, Kenny D, Blaton, Burnett D, Huisman W, Plebani M, Queraltó JM, Zérah S, van Lieshout J. Usefulness of EC4 Essential criteria for Quality Systems of medical Laboratories as Guideline to the ISO 15189 and ISO 17025 Documents. Clin Chem Med Lab 2000; **38:** 1057-64 (www.uni-oldenberg.de/ec4/).

Jansen, RTP, Blaton V, Burnett D, Huisman W, Queraltó JM, Zérah S, Allman B. Additional essential criteria for quality systems of medical laboratories. Clin Chem Lab Med 1998; **36:** 249-52 (www.uni-oldenberg.de/ec4/).

CHAPTER 3 – QUALITY MANAGEMENT FOR THE MEDICAL LABORATORY

*ISO 9000:2000 Quality management systems – Fundamentals and vocabulary.

*ISO 9004:2000 Quality management systems – Guidelines for performance improvements.

Guidelines for quality systems in medical laboratories, National Pathology Accreditation Advisory Council (NPAAC), Canberra, Australia, 2001 (www.health.gov.au/npaac).

CHAPTER 4 – ORGANISATION AND MANAGEMENT RESPONSIBILITY

Audit Commission. The Pathology Services – A Management Review. HMSO, London, 1991.

Code of Conduct/Accountability for NHS Boards, Department of Health (UK) 1994.

Draft Standards for Pathology Laboratories, National Pathology Accreditation Advisory Council, Canberra, Australia, 2001 (www.health.gov.au/npaac).

Dybkaer R, Jordal R, Jorgensen PT et al. A quality manual for the clinical laboratory - including elements of a quality system. Proposed guidelines. Scand J Clin Lab Invest 1993; **53 (Suppl 212):** 60-82.

Guidance Documents Available from Accreditation Bodies for the Preparation of Laboratory Quality Manuals, ILAC-14 1996 (www.ilac.org).

ISO 10013:1995(E). Guidelines for developing quality manuals.

ISO/IEC 15189:2002 Medical Laboratories – Particular requirements for quality and competence, Annex C, Ethics in Laboratory Medicine.

Queraltó JM. The EC4 Quality Manual Model. Clin Chim Acta 2001; **309:** 127-36.

Sanders GT, Kelly AM, Breur J, Kohse K, Mocarelli P, Sachs C. The European Register for Clinical Chemists. Eur J Clin Chem Clin Biochem 1997; **35:** 795-6.

Standards of business conduct for NHS Staff, NHS Management Executive HSG (93)5 1993.

CHAPTER 5 – A QUALITY MANAGEMENT SYSTEM AND DOCUMENTATION

Retention of Laboratory Records and Diagnostic Material. Commonwealth Department of Health NPAAC, Canberra, Australia, Draft 2nd edition 2001. (www.health.gov.au/npaac).

The Retention and Storage of Pathological Records and Archives. Report of the Working Party of the Royal College of Pathologists and the Institute of Biomedical Science, 2nd Edition 1999 (www.rcpath.org.uk).

Use and Disclosure of Health Data Guidance on the Application of the Data Protection Act 1998, 2002.

CHAPTER 6 – PERSONNEL

Code of Practice on Discliplinary and Grievances Procedures, ACAS 2000 (www.acas.org.uk).

Employment Handbook, The A-Z of work, ACAS 2001 (www.acas.org.uk).

Good Medical Practice in Pathology. RCPath, 2001 (www.rcpath.org.uk).

Substandard professional performance: guidance for Trusts and pathologists. The Royal College of Pathologists (RCPath), 2002. (www.rcpath.org.uk).

The Internet: A Writer's Guide. Jane Dournier, A & C Black (Publishers) Ltd, London, 2000.

Working Together – the ACAS standard, Advisory, Conciliation and Arbitration service. (ACAS), 2000 (www.acas.org.uk).

CHAPTER 7 – PREMISES AND ENVIRONMENT

5 steps to risk assessment. 1998 HSE, UK. (www.hse.gov.uk).

A guide to risk assessment requirements – Common provision in health and safety law. 1999 HSE, UK. (www.hse.gov.uk).

A short guide to Personal protective Equipment at Work Regulations. 1996, HSE, UK (www.hse.gov.uk).

Categorisation of biological agents according to hazard and categories of containment (out of print – to be replaced by Biological Agents – Managing the risks 2003), Health and Safety Commission, Advisory Committee on Dangerous Pathogens. HSE Books, Sudbury, UK.

Clinical Laboratory Safety; Approved Guideline 1996. NCCLS Document GP17-A.

Clinical Laboratory Waste Management; Approved Guideline 1993. NCCLS Document GP5-A.

College of American Pathologists (CAP), Laboratory General Checklist: section on laboratory safety. 2001 (www.cap.org).

Directive 90/679/EEC on the protection of workers from the risks related to exposure to biological agents at work, 1990.

Directive 98/24/EC on the protection of the health and safety of workers from the risks related to chemical agents at work, 1998.

Everyone's guide to RIDDOR, 1995; Reporting of injuries, diseases and dangerous occurrences regulations, HSE, UK (www.hse.gov.uk).

Facilities for mortuary and post-mortem room services, HBN 20, NHS Estates, Department of Health, 2001 (www.nhsestates.gov.uk).

Five steps to risk assessment, 1994; A step by step guide to a safer and healthier workplace, HSE, UK.

Guidelines for approved pathology collection centres, NPAAC, Canberra, Australia, 2000 (www.health.gov.au/npaac).

Healthcare Waste Minimisation, a compendium of good practice. NHS Estates, Department of Health, 2000 (www.nhsestates.gov.uk).

HIV and the Practice of Pathology, Report of the Working Party of the Royal College of Pathologists. RCPath 1995 (www.rcpath.org).

Implementing a Needlestick and Sharps Injury Prevention Program in a Clinical Laboratory; A Report 2002. NCCLS Document X3-R.

ISO 14001:1996 Environmental management systems – Specifications with guidance for use.

ISO/DIS 15190 (Sept 2001) Medical Laboratories – Safety management.

Laboratory Assessment Checklist, Blood Banks and Transfusion Services. NPAAC, Canberra, Australia, 1995 (www.health.gov.au/npaac).

Managing health and safety, Five steps to success. Health and Safety Executive (HSE) UK, 1998 (www.hse.gov.uk).

Manual handling: Manual Handling Operations Regulations 1992, Guidance on Regulations. HSE Books, Sudbury, UK. (www.hse.gov.uk).

Mortland KK, Mortland D. Does Your Laboratory Meet Code. Clinical Leadership & Management Review. July/August 2000; 160-5.

Mortland KK, Mortland D. Practical Lessons in Laboratory Planning. Clinical Leadership & Management Review. Nov/Dec 2001; 388-90 (www.mortlanddesign.com).

OHSAS 18001:1999 Occupational health and safety management systems – Specification.

OHSAS 18002:2000 Occupational health and safety management systems – Guidelines for the implementation of OHSAS 18001.

prEN 13641 Elimination or reduction of risk of infection related to in vitro diagnostic reagents.

Procedures for the Collection of Diagnostic Blood Specimens by Venipuncture; Approved Standard – Fourth Edition 1998 NCCLS Document H3-A4.

Protection of Laboratory Workers from Occupationally acquired Infections; Approved Guideline – Second Edition. 2002 NCCLS Document M29-A2.

Safe working and the prevention of infection in clinical laboratories – model rules for staff and visitors, 1991; Health Services Advisory Committee, HSE Books, Sudbury, UK.

Safe working and the prevention of infection in clinical laboratories, 1991; Health Services Advisory Committee, Safety in Health Service Laboratories, Health and Safety Commission, HSE Books, Sudbury, UK.

Tackling work-related stress, A guide for employees. 2001 HSE, UK. (www.hse.gov.uk).

The management design and operation of microbiological containment laboratories. 2001; Health and Safety Commission, Advisory Committee on Dangerous Pathogens, HSE Books, Sudbury, UK.

The Reporting of Injuries, Diseases and Dangerous Occurrence Regulations 1995: Guidance for employers in the healthcare sector, Health Services Sheet 1. 1998 HSE, UK. (www.hse.gov.uk).

Wayfinding, Effective wayfinding and signing systems – Guidance for healthcare facilities. NHS Estates, Department of Health, 1999 (www.nhsestates.gov.uk).

Working with VDUs. 1998 HSE, UK. (www.hse.gov.uk).

Workplace, Health, Safety and Welfare, a short guide for managers. HSE, UK, 1997 (www.hse.gov.uk).

CHAPTER 8 – EQUIPMENT AND DIAGNOSTIC SYSTEMS (IVDS), AND DATA AND INFORMATION SYSTEMS

Anderson R, Clinical System Security: Interim Guidelines. Brit Med J 1996; **312:** 109-11.

Bremond J, Plebani M. IVD industry role for quality and accreditation in medical laboratories. Clin Chim Acta 2001; **309:** 167-71.

Directive 98/79/EC on in vitro diagnostic medical devices, 1998.

EN 13612:2002 Performance evaluation of in vitro diagnostic medical devices.

EN 375:2001 Information supplied by the manufacturer with in vitro diagnostic reagents for professional use.

EN 376:2002 Information supplied by the manufacturer with in vitro diagnostics for self-testing.

EN 591:2001 Instructions for use for in vitro diagnostic instruments for professional use.

EN 592:2002 Instructions for use for in vitro diagnostic instruments for self-testing.

Gogates, G D, Excel 97 Data security 2001 (www.fasor.com).

Gogates, G D, Software Validation in Accredited Laboratories, A Practical Guide 2001 (www.fasor.com).

ISO/IEC 15189:2002 Medical Laboratories – Particular requirements for quality and competence, Annex B Laboratory Information Systems (LIS).

Management and Use of IVD Point of Care Test devices. MDA Device Bulletin 2002(03) 2002 (www.medical-devices.gov.uk).

Management of In Vitro Diagnostic Medical Devices. MDA Device Bulletin 2002(02) 2002 (www.medical-devices.gov.uk).

Medical Device and Equipment Management for Hospital and Community-based Organisations. Medical Devices Agency (MDA), Device Bulletin 9801 1998 – Supplement 1 Checks and tests for newly delivered medical devices 1999- Supplement 2 Guidance on the sale, Transfer of Ownership and Disposal of Used Medical Devices (www.medical-devices.gov.uk).

The application of the principles of GLP to computerised systems 'Environmental Monograph No 116, 1995 OECD Paris (www.oecd.org).

CHAPTER 9 – PRE- AND POST-EXAMINATION PROCESSES

Blood Gas Preanalytical Considerations: Specimen Collection, Calibration, and Controls; Approved Guideline 1993 NCCLS Document C27-A.

Clinical Laboratory Safety; Approved Guideline 1996 NCCLS Document GP17-A.

Clinical Laboratory Technical Procedure Manuals – Fourth Edition; Approved Guideline 2002 NCCLS Document GP2-A4.

Clinical Laboratory Waste Management – Second Edition; Approved Guideline 2002 NCCLS Document GP5-A2.

Collection, Transport and Processing of Blood Specimens for Coagulation Testing and Performance of Coagulation Assays; Approved Guideline – Third Edition 1998 NCCLS Document H21-A3.

College of American Pathologists, Protocols for reporting histopathology. 2002 (www.cap.org).

College of American Pathologists, Reporting on Cancer Specimens: Protocols and Case Summaries. CAP: Northfield, IL, 1999.

Confidentiality: Protecting and Providing Information, General Medical Council, London 2000.

Convention for the protection of human rights and dignity of the human being with regard to the application of biology and medicine: Convention on Human Rights and Biomedicine. Council of Europe, European Treaty Series No 164, 1997 (www.europa.eu.int).

COSHH in Laboratories, Second edition. The Royal Society of Chemistry 1996.

Cote RA, Rothwell DJ, Palotay JL, Becket RS, Brochu L. (eds), The Systemized Nomenclature of Medicine: SNOMED® International. College of American Pathologists, Northfield, IL, 1993.

Data Protection Act 1998. London: The Stationery Office Ltd, 1998.

Devices for Collection of Skin Puncture Blood Specimens – Second Edition; Approved Guideline 1990 NCCLS Document H14-A2.

Evacuated Tubes for Blood Specimen Collection – Third Edition; Approved Standard 1991 NCCLS Document H1-A3.

Examination of the body after death – Information about post-mortem examination for relatives, Royal College of Pathologists UK, 2000 (www.rcpath.org).

Examining the body after death – Information for relatives about post-mortems, Chesterfield and North Derbyshire Royal Hospital, NHS Trust 2002.

Good practice in consent implementation guide – consent to examination treatment, DoH, UK 2001 (www.doh.gov.uk).

Guidelines for data communication, NPAAC, Canberra, Australia, 1998 (www.health.gov.au/npaac).

Guidelines for the preparation of laboratory manuals (including Laboratory Handbooks), NPAAC, Canberra, Australia, 1986 (reprinted 1999) (www.health.gov.au/npaac).

Guidelines for the Safe Transport of Infectious substances. WHO/EMC/97.3, WHO 1997 (www.who.int).

How to Define, Determine, and Utilize Reference Intervals in the Clinical Laboratory; Approved Guideline 1995 NCCLS Document C28-A.

IATA Dangerous Goods Regulation, 39th Edition, 1998.

Information on the transport of pathology specimens, NPAAC, Canberra, Australia (www.health.gov.au/npaac).

NCCLS Selecting and Evaluating a Referral Laboratory; Approved Guideline 1998 NCCLS Document GP9-A.

Pneumatic air tube transports systems, Design considerations and Good Practice guide and Management policy. NHS Estates, UK, 1995.

Procedures for the Collection of Arterial Blood Specimens; Approved Standard – Third Edition (1999) NCCLS Document H11-A3.

Procedures for the Collection of Diagnostic Blood Specimens by Skin Puncture; Approved Standard – Fourth Edition 1999 NCCLS Document H4-A4.

Procedures for the Handling and Processing of Blood Specimens; Approved Guideline – Second Edition 1999 NCCLS Document H18-A2.

Protecting and Using Patient Information – A Manual for Caldicott Guardians, NHS Executive (www.doh.gov.uk).

Routine Urinalysis and Collection, Transportation, and Preservation of Urine Specimens – Second Edition; Approved Guideline 2001 NCCLS Document GP16-A2.

Safe use of pneumatic air tube transport systems for pathology specimens, HSE Information Sheet, HSE, UK, 1999 (www.hse.gov.uk).

Safety in Health Service Laboratories: The labelling, transport and reception of samples 1986; Health Services Advisory Committee, HSE Books, Sudbury, UK.

Selecting and Evaluating a Referral Laboratory; Tentative Guideline 1991, NCCLS Document GP9-T.

Sharp S, Cummins D, Halloran S, Donaldson M, Turnbull L. Explosions may occur if dry ice is placed in airtight transport container. Brit Med J 2001; 322: 434.

SNOMED® Clinical terms, From development to Evaluation and Implementation. NHS Information Authority 2001 (www.coding.nhsia.nhs.uk).

The Caldicott Committee: Report on the review of patient-identifiable information. London, NHS Executive, UK 1997.

The Removal, Retention and use of Human Organs and Tissue from Post-mortem Examinations. Advice from the Chief Medical Officer, DoH UK, 2001 (www.doh.gov.uk).

The Royal College of Pathologists' advice relating to the ownership, storage and release of pathology results. Royal College of Pathologists UK 2001 (www.rcpath.org).

Use and Disclosure of Health Data, Guidance on the Application of the Data Protection Act 1998. 2002 (www.informationcommisioner.gov.uk).

User Manual, Respiratory and Systemic Infection Laboratory, Central Public Health Laboratory, PHLS UK 2002 (www.phls.org.uk).

CHAPTER 10 – EXAMINATION PROCESSES

A Framework for NCCLS Evaluation Protocols; A Report, 2002, NCCLS Document EP19-R.

Burnett D. Accreditation and point-of-care testing. Ann Clin Biochem 2000; **37:** 241-3.

Directive 98/24/EC on the protection of the health and safety of workers from the risks related to chemical agents at work.

EN 12322:1999 In vitro diagnostic medical devices – Culture media for microbiology – Performance criteria for culture media.

EN 12376:1999 In vitro diagnostic medical devices – Information supplied by the manufacturer with in vitro diagnostic reagents for staining in biology.

EN 13641:2002 Elimination of risk of infection related to in vitro diagnostic reagents.

Strategies to Set Global Analytical Quality Specifications in Laboratory Medicine, Scand J Clin Lab Invest 1999; **59:** 475-585.

Estimation of the Total Analytical Error for Clinical Laboratory Methods; Proposed Guideline 2002 NCCLS Document EP21-P.

Evaluation of the Linearity of Quantitative Analytical Methods; Proposed Guideline – Second Edition 2001 NCCLS Document EP6-P2.

Fraser CG, Kallner A, Kenny D, Hyltoft Petersen P. Introduction: Strategies to set global quality specifications in laboratory medicine. Scand J Clin Lab Invest 1999; **59:** 477-8.

Goldschimdt HMJ. Postanalytical factors and their influence on analytical quality specifications Scand J Clin Lab Invest 1999; **59:** 551-4.

Guder WG. Preanalytical factors and their influence on analytical quality specifications. Scand J Clin Lab Invest 1999; **59:** 545-50.

Guide to the expression of uncertainty in measurement issued by BIPM, IEC, IFCC, ISO, IUPAC, IUPAP and OIML, ISO 1995.

Guidelines for the performance of the pathology surgical cutup. NPAAC, Canberra, Australia, 2001 (www.health.gov.au/npaac).

Guidelines for the preparation of laboratory manuals. NPAAC, Canberra, Australia, 1986 (reprinted 1999) (www.health.gov.au/npaac).

Histopathology of limited or no value. RCPath Histopathology Working Group 2001 (www.rcpath.org).

Investigation of urine, PHLS Standard Operating Procedure B.SOP 41 Central Public Health Laboratory, PHLS UK 2002 (www.phls.org.uk).

Kallner A, Uncertainty in measurement – Introduction and examples from laboratory medicine. eJIFCC **12(4):** 2001 (www.ifcc.org/ejifccc).

Kenny D, Fraser CG, Hyltoft Petersen P, Kallner A. Consensus agreement. Scand J Clin Lab Invest 1999; **59:** 585.

Method Comparison and Bias Estimation Using Patient Samples; Approved Guideline 1995 NCCLS Document EP9-A.

Point-of-Care Testing ed. Price CP, Hicks JM. AACC, 1999 (www.aaccdirect.org)

Quantifying Uncertainty in Analytical Measurement. EURACHEM/CITAC Guide, QUAM:2000.P1, 2nd Edition 2000 (www.eurachem.ul.pt).

Requirements for gynaecological (cervical) cytology. NPAAC, Canberra, Australia, 1997 (www.health.gov.au/npaac).

The Fitness for Purpose of Analytical Methods, A Laboratory Guide to Method validation and related Topics. EURACHEM Guide, 1st Edition 1999 (www.eurachem.ul.pt).

Evidence and diagnostics. Bandolier Extra, February 2002 (www.ebandolier.com).

Accreditation for microbiological laboratories EA-4/10 European Co-operation for Accreditation 2002 (www.european-accreditation.org).

CHAPTER 11 – EVALUATION AND QUALITY IMPROVEMENT

Criteria for the Assessment of External Quality Assurance Programs, Vol.1,

Clinical Biochemistry, Haematology, Microbiology Vol.2, Transfusion Serology, Anatomical Pathology, and Cytology Vol.3, Immunology and Cytogenetics and Guidelines for Gynaecological (Cervical) Cytology.NPAAC, Canberra, Australia, (www.health.gov.au/npaac).

Donabedian A. Evaluating the Quality of Medical Care. Millbank Memorial Fund Quarterly 1996; 44:166-206.

Goldie DJ. Accreditation of external quality assessment schemes in the United Kingdom. Clin Chim Acta 2001; **309:** 179-81.

ILAC-G13-2000: Guidelines for the requirements for the competence of providers of proficiency testing Schemes (www.ilac.org).

Internal Audits and Management Review for Laboratories EAL-G3 European cooperation for Accreditation 1996.

ISO 9004:2000 Quality management systems – Guidelines for performance improvements.

ISO Guide 43-1: 1997 Proficiency testing by interlaboratory comparisons – Part 1: Development and operation of proficiency testing Schemes.

ISO Guide 43-2: 1997 Proficiency testing by interlaboratory comparisons – Part 2: Selection and use of proficiency testing Schemes by laboratory accreditation bodies.

Laboratory-Related Measures of Patient Outcomes: An Introduction, ed. Bissell MG. AACC 2000 (www.aaccdirect.org).

Maxwell RJ. Quality Assessment in Health. Brit Med J 1984; **288:** 1470-2.

Plebani M. Role of inspectors in external review mechanisms: criteria for selection, training and appraisal. Clin Chim Acta 2001; **309:** 147-54.

Sciacovelli L, Secchiero S, Zardo L, Plebani M. External Quality Assessment Schemes: need for recognised requirements. Clin Chim Acta 2001; **309:** 183-99.

UK NEQAS Assessment of Clinical Interpretation, UK NEQAS (Birmingham), 2002 (www.ukneqas.org.uk).

Waise A, Plebani M. Which surrogate marker can be used to assess the effectiveness of the laboratory and its contribution to clinical outcome? Ann Clin Biochem 2001; **38:** 589-95.

Index